Vegan Diet

Low Fodmap Diet Vegetarian and Delicious Recipes

(Top 50 Low Carb Vegan Recipes for Beginners)

Kenny Brown

Published by Robert Satterfield Publishing House

© **Kenny Brown**

All Rights Reserved

Vegan Diet: Low Fodmap Diet Vegetarian and Delicious Recipes (Top 50 Low Carb Vegan Recipes for Beginners)

ISBN 978-1-989787-32-8

All rights reserved. No part of this guide may be reproduced in any form without permission in writing from the publisher except in the case of brief quotations embodied in critical articles or reviews.

Legal & Disclaimer

The information contained in this book is not designed to replace or take the place of any form of medicine or professional medical advice. The information in this book has been provided for educational and entertainment purposes only.

The information contained in this book has been compiled from sources deemed reliable, and it is accurate to the best of the Author's knowledge; however, the Author cannot guarantee its accuracy and validity and cannot be held liable for any errors or omissions. Changes are periodically made to this book. You must consult your doctor or get professional medical advice before using any of the suggested remedies, techniques, or information in this book.

TABLE OF CONTENT

Part 1 1

Introduction 2

Chapter 1 - What It Means To Be Vegan? 4

Chapter 2 - History Of Veganism 9

Chapter 3 - Veganism's Impact On The Environment 12

Chapter 4 - Before Going Vegan 20

Chapter 5 - Healthy Eating As A Vegan 27

Chapter 6 - Other Vegan Living Aspects 34

Conclusion 36

Part 2 37

Introduction 38

Chapter 1: Breakfast Choices 43

BEVERAGES 43

Apple Pear Cider In The Slow Cooker 43

Dirty Chai 45

Iced Thai Tea Concentrate 47

Other Breakfast Dishes 49

Blueberry Banana Muffins 49

Crepes 51

Pancakes With Bananas 52

Pancakes With Sweet Potatoes 55

Quinoa & Strawberry Infused Cereal 58

Scrambled Tofu 60

Veggie Omelet In The Crock Pot 61

Chapter 2: Lunchtime Favorites 64

Butternut Squash & Macaroni In The Crock Pot 64

Cauliflower Alfredo With Parmesan 66

Corn Risotto In The Slow Cooker 69

Curried Carrot Fritters 70

Kale & Sweet Potato Hash 73

Quinoa Tabbouleh 75

Shepherd's Pie With Lentils 77

Vegan Meatloaf With Gravy 79

Vegetable Curry 82

Chapter 3: Healthy Soups & Stews 85

Soups 85

Butternut Squash Soup In The Slow Cooker 85

Coconut Curry Chickpea Lentil Soup 87

Corn And Red Pepper Chowder 89

Homestyle Chickpea Noodle Soup... 91

Kale Soup 94

Lentil And Apricot Soup In A Slow Cooker 96

Stews & Chilis.. 98

Chickpea And Sweet Potato Chili 98

3-Bean Sweet Potato Chili 101

Tomato-Curry Lentil Stew 103

Sides Or Veggies.. 105

Baked Spaghetti Squash.. 105

Bbq Baked Beans 108

Tofu Noodles... 111

Chapter 4: Delicious Sandwiches & Salads 114

Salads.. 114

Caesar Salad.. 114

Chickpea Tomatoes & Peppers Salad 116

Sauerkraut Salad... 117

3-Bean Salad 119

Chapter 5: Dips, Snacks, & Appetizers................................ 121

Dips & Spreads 121

Barbecue Sauce 121

Black Olive Fig & Tapenade With Rosemary 122

Sour Cream 124

Taco Seasoning 125

White Bean Hummus 127

Snacks 128

Banana Cookies 128

Cashew & Dates Dessert 130

Double-Chocolate, Almond Chia Seed Granola Bars 131

Oatmeal Energy Bars 134

Appetizers 136

Mushroom Bruschetta Crostini 136

White Bean Bruschetta 138

Chapter 6: Desserts 140

Pumpkin & Apple Dessert 140

Pumpkin Bread 142

Raw Strawberry Pie 144

Smoothies 146

Banana Pineapple & Nutty Smoothie 146

Blueberry & Lemonade Smoothie 147

Cherry 149

Smoothie... 149

Chia Banana & Green Tea Smoothie.................................. 150

Matcha Coconut Smoothie 152

Orange Juice Goji Berries Smoothie 153

Conclusion 155

About The Author 156

Part 1

Introduction

I want to thank you and congratulate you for downloading my book.

This book contains proven steps and strategies on how to transition from a carnivorous or omnivorous diet to a nutritious and delicious plant-based diet and how this transition impacts the environment.

Let's not pretend that going vegan is easy. It takes courage to go vegan. Imagine passing over the charcoal-broiled cheeseburger and reaching for a veggie burger instead. But as you read my book, you will be convinced that the reasons why you should practice the vegan lifestyle are well worth it. Inside are tips and tricks to make the vegan diet transition easier. You will also learn more about veganism, its history, its benefits to your health, and how adhering to it can benefit the environment.

Thanks again for downloading this book, I hope you enjoy it!

Chapter 1 - What it Means to be Vegan?

Being a vegan is not just about eating plant-based foods and shunning those that are derived from animals. It's also a lifestyle. As much as possible, veganism, which is an extreme form of vegetarianism, seeks to exclude all forms of exploitation (including cruelty) to animals for clothing, food or any other purpose.

Strict veganism forbids the use of food and non-food animal products. Animal products contain Vitamin B12, so vegans must take a vitamin supplement or B12-fortified food to get its recommended amount. While American vegetarianism has deviated from its religious and philosophical roots, veganism is still tethered to the animal rights movement.

Vegans can be as lax or strict as they want to be when it comes to choosing food. A good reference, the website of the International Vegetarian Union (ivu.org), contains vegan-friendly reminders on cereals with animal-derived glycerin, baking pans coated with animal fat and bone charcoal-refined sugar. There's the so-called raw veganism, which is a veganism offshoot wherein adherents eat only uncooked food. Go one step further and you have'mono meals,'which is the notion that the stomach must only digest one kind of food at any given time.

What Vegans Eat

Being vegan doesn't mean that the food choices are limited. As you go vegan, your perspective on food alsochanges. You'll discover a new world of exciting flavors and foods that you likely would never have found if you had continued your traditional diet. A vegan diet is diverse and contains all kinds of vegetables, fruits, seeds, grains, nuts, pulses and beans. All these foods have multiple combinations so you'll never be bored.

From cake to curry, pizzas to pies, you can prepare all your favorite foods and make them suitable to a vegan diet. All that you have to do is to prepare them with plant-based ingredients.

Vegans never exploit animals. Compassion for animals is the primary reason why many individuals seek a vegan lifestyle. While animal-derived ingredients can be found in everything from clothing and accessories to bathroom items, there are readily available and affordable alternatives nowadays to almost everything.

Health Benefits of Going Vegan

Vegan diets are known to provide a lot of benefits, including a reduced risk of diabetes, premature death and cancer. However, you need to realize that not all vegan diets are the same. This is due to the abundance of vegan junk food, which can include sweet treats, salty snacks and starchy food items.

You can discern healthy vegan foods from vegan junk food. When you subscribe to a healthy vegan diet, you tend to eat more fiber, thus decreasing your risk of developing colorectal cancer. Vegans are also more likely to consume at least seven servings of fruits and vegetables a day, which means you have a 33% reduced premature death risk–compared to meat-eating individuals.

With the wide array of simple and tasty vegan meals that are packed with vegetables and fruits, it's not surprising that vegans reap such benefits. Vegans also benefit from eating low-calorie meals. When compared to other dietary groups, vegans have lower BMIs (body mass index), have lower percentages of body fat and are leaner.

It also means that vegans are not as likely to get weight-related conditions like diabetes. Vegan males also have a reduced prostate cancer risk. In general, vegans have reduced risk of heart attacks. They also have lower mortality rates, blood pressure and cholesterol.

A study done by experts at Oxford University's Oxford Martin School found that–by 2050–adoption of plant-based diets by most people would prevent 8.1

million premature deaths a year. It may be due to several factors including the reduction of processed food and red meat, which the WHO (World Health Organization) has considered carcinogenic because of the colorectal cancer risk.

It's interesting to note that that there are benefits of going vegan that you can almost feel immediately. Many vegans experience clearer skin, increased energy, stronger nails and hair, reduced allergy symptoms, and relief from the pain of PMS and migraine headaches.

You will also feel a general sense of well being, knowing that your current lifestyle limits environmental damage and reduces animal suffering. Don't be guilty if you tend to overeat on that vegan cupcake; you're doing an excellent job. Know that your chances of living a healthier and longer life are raised by eating plenty of whole grains, green leafy vegetables and other nutritious foods every day.

Chapter 2 - History of Veganism

Although the term 'veganism' was first used in 1944, the concept of avoiding animal flesh can be traced back to ancient eastern Mediterranean and Indian societies. Around 500 BCE, Pythagoras of Samos, a Greek mathematician and philosopher, first mentioned vegetarianism. Pythagoras, in addition to his right triangle theorem, promoted benevolence among humans and all other species.

Followers of Hinduism, Buddhism and Jainism also advocated for vegetarianism. They believed that human beings must not inflict pain on animals. However, the meatless advocacy never caught on in the Western world, although it did occasionally pop up during religious revivals and health crazes.

The Ephrata Cloister, a religious sect established in Pennsylvania, promoted both vegetarianism and celibacy. Jeremy Bentham —an 18th century utilitarian philosopher –believed that animal suffering was equal to human suffering. He equated the notion of human superiority to racism.

In 1847, the first vegetarian society was established in England. Three years later, the creator of Graham crackers–Presbyterian minister Rev. Sylvester Graham–founded the American Vegetarian Society. He and his Grahamites (his followers) adhered to Graham's instructions for a noble life: abstinence, vegetarianism, frequent bathing and temperance.

In November of 1944, British woodworker Donald Watson stated that, since vegetarians ate eggs and dairy, he would use a new word 'vegan' to describe people who shunned those things. In 1943, tuberculosis had been found in 40% of the country's cows, and Watson used that situation advantageously. He claimed that veganism protected people from contaminated food.

Three months after coining the word 'vegan,' Watson explained how to pronounce the word. By the time he died in 2005 at the age of 95, there were 250,000 self-described vegans in the United Kingdom and 2 million in the United States.

Chapter 3 - Veganism's Impact on the Environment

There are many reasons why you should go vegan. People switch to the vegan lifestyle to improve their health. Well-planned, plant-based diets are rich in calcium, iron, protein and other important minerals and vitamins. Plant-based diets are packed with antioxidants, high in fiber, and low in saturated fat. Such diets also help mitigate certain contemporary health issues like cancer, diabetes, heart disease and obesity.

Another reason for going vegan is that it benefits the animal world. Avoiding animal products is one of the most apparent ways to fight back against animal exploitation and animal cruelty.

Others also switch to veganism for human health and the health of our planet. Veganism is the sustainable choice when it comes to caring for the planet, and therefore a plant-based diet can be a more sustainable way to feed a family. A vegan diet only needs 1/3 of the land needed to support a dairy-and-meat diet.

With rising global water and food insecurity as a resultof various socio-economic and environmental problems, there's never been a better time to switch to a more sustainable lifestyle. Avoiding animal products is one way to reduce the strain on natural resources and food. It is also a good way to battle against inefficient food systems that disproportionately affect the world's poorest people.

Caring for the environment is also one of the reasons why some people decide to switch to veganism. From bicycling to work to recycling household garbage, everyone is aware of how important it is to follow a green lifestyle. An effective way to care for the environment is to lower your carbon footprint by absolutely avoiding animal products.

Plus, raising animals for food requires tremendous amounts of energy, feed, land

and water. And this practice causes animals unimaginable levels of pain and suffering.

Climate Change

According to a Worldwatch Institute report, approximately 51% of greenhouse gas emissions are a result of animal agriculture. The United Nations states that a concerted global shift to a vegan diet is necessary in fighting the worst effects of climate change.

Water Use

It takes a lot of water to clean dirty factory farms, grow crops for animals to consume, and give animals water for drinking. Just one milking cow can consume more than 50 gallons of water in a single day, sometimes as much as 100 gallons on a hot day. The math isn't pretty. The result is that it takes 683 gallons of water to produce one gallon of milk.

In another example, it takes more than 2,400 gallons of water to produce one pound of beef. By comparison, 244 gallons of water are needed to produce one pound of tofu. By going vegan, a person can save approximately 219,000 gallons of water a year. Imagine the rest of the human population doing this. The world would certainly be a better place with lots of potable and clean water for all.

Land Use

It is inefficient to use land to grow crops to feed animals. It entails nearly 20 times less land to feed a person on a vegan diet than it does to support a meat-eater since the crops are directly consumed, instead feeding them to animals.

According to the United Nations Convention to Combat Desertification, it takes around 10 pounds of grain to make only one pound of meat. In the U.S. alone, around 56 million acres of land are utilized to grow hay for livestock, while only 4 million acres grow plants for human consumption.

Over 90 percent of the Amazon rainforest cleared since the 1970s is used for livestock grazing. Moreover, one of the primary crops grown in cleared rainforest acreage is soybeans, which is for animal feeding. It would certainly be better to feed these soybeans to humans instead of animals. The impact of this move to the environment would be lesser.

Pollution

In the United States, animals raised for food produce more excrement than the country's human population. According to the U.S. EPA (Environmental Protection Agency), animals on factory farms in the U.S. produce around 500 million tons of manure annually. As there are no processing plants for animal sewage, the manure is stored in waste 'lagoons' or they get sprayed over fields.

Runoff from livestock grazing and factory farms is one of the main causes of lake and river pollution. The EPA notes that viruses and bacteria can be transported by the runoff and that groundwater can get contaminated.

Factory farms evade water pollution limits by spraying liquid manure into the air, creating wind-borne mists. People who live near such farms inhale the pathogens and the toxins from the sprayed manure. A California State Senate report cites studies that indicate "animal waste lagoons emit toxic airborne substances that can cause irritation, immune, neurochemical, and inflammatory problems in humans."

Oceans

Just as factory farms pollute the land, commercial fishing methods like long-lining and bottom trawling often sweep and ravage the ocean floor of life. Such methods also destroy coral reefs in the process. These fishing methods also kill thousands of sea turtles, sharks, dolphins and other so called 'bycatch' marine species.

And farmed fish aren't much better for the planet, either. Fish farms along the coast release parasites, antibiotics, feces and non-native fish into highly sensitive marine ecosystems. Since most farmed fish are carnivores, they require lots of wild-caught fish as food. For example, it takes approximately three pounds of feed to produce one pound of farmed fish.

Social and Environmental Impact

The vegan diet's social and environmental impact is staggering. Anywhere from80 to 90 percent of the planet's crops are used as livestock feed. Instead, these crops could easily feed impoverished people around the world if more people adopted a vegan diet.

What you choose to eat vastly impacts others and the rest of the world. You can help improve your life and the lives of others –and benefit the environment in the process–by switchingto a vegan diet. It's not just about what you give up, it's also about what you get.

A vegan diet comes with many benefits, including living longer, saving money, and living a life that's in line with your values. You're not just talking the talk. Following the vegan way of life is walking the walk. You get the satisfaction of knowing that you are not harming any animals with your lifestyle, right down to the very shoes you wear and car you drive. Following a vegan diet and lifestyle has less of an impact on the world's increasingly scarce natural resources.

Chapter 4 - Before Going Vegan

Once followed primarily by peace-loving hippies, interest in veganism has since become high, thanks to the advocacies of celebrities like Alicia Silverstone, Bill Clinton, Beyoncé, Jay Z, and others. But before going vegan and jumping onboard the no-dairy-meat-or-eggs bandwagon, you should be aware of a few things.

B12 Supplements

Vitamin B12 is naturally found in animal products. If you decide to go vegan, you may want find a B12 supplement and research foods fortified with B12. B12 helps keep the body's blood and nerve cells healthy. B12 also helps in creating DNA, which means that any deficiency in this vitamin can lead to weakness, tiredness, loss of appetite, constipation, nerve problems, weight loss and depression. To determine if you need to take more B12, ask your doctor to run a blood test.

Iron Supplements

Iron has two forms: non-heme and heme. Comprising about 40% of the iron in animal products, heme is absorbed easily by the body. The diets of vegans only have non-heme, which is not easily absorbed. Therefore, you may have to take more iron if you want the same benefits.

Good natural iron sources for vegans include dried raisins, sunflower seeds, legumes and leafy dark greens. Plus, foods rich in Vitamin C (broccoli, citrus and red peppers) help in iron absorption.

Questions from Family and Friends

According to Julieanna Hever, a plant-based dietitian, people can be sensitive regarding their diets, especially when their beliefs about food are challenged. She adds that the best way to lessen conflict is to affirm that you are switching to veganism for your own reasons that seem to work to your benefit. It's about you, and you don't have to feel the need to defend your choice to anyone.

New Protein Sources

Every meal must have protein, which is life's building block. Proteins break down into amino acids, promoting cell repair and growth. The Institute of Medicine states that adults must have a minimum of 0.8 grams of protein every day for each kg of body mass. Vegan protein sources, among many others, include soy, seitan, nuts, quinoa and beans.

Junk Food does not Replace Animal Products

Substituting meat with pasta, packaged or processed foodsand white bread sets you up for vegan diet failure. It's not a good idea to substitute animal products (rich in minerals, vitamins, and protein) with processed foods that contain little nutritional value aside from calories.

Limit the Soy

While scientists are figuring out soy's effects on heart health and cancer, one thing is for sure: eating too much of vegan 'meat' produced from soy is arguably worse in terms of nutrition than eating high-quality animal products. Carefully read the labels as meat substitutes are often highly processed and loaded with preservatives and sodium. The healthiest soy sources are edamame, soy milk, tofu, tempeh and miso.

Ease Into It

You don't become a vegan overnight, as going vegan takes a lot of work and time. Begin by consuming more plant-based foods. At the same time, cut back on non-organic animal products andrefined, processed foods. What's important is making slow changes and assessing how you feel.

Learn to Read Labels

If you are set to go vegan, it's important to verify ingredients by checking food labels. Just because a food product is not apparently non-vegan doesn't mean it is right for a vegan diet. Milk-based whey and casein are found in most granolas, breads, and cereal bars, while tallow (suet) and gelatin are taken from meat. You should also be mindful of Natural Red 4 (aka cochineal, cochineal extract, or carmine), which is a food coloring from dried female beetles' bodies.

Feeling Happier

A 2012 Nutrition Journal study states that, compared to vegetarian diets, vegan diets have more arachidonic acid, which can promote neurological shifts that help improve moods. Apparently it's not just animals that will be happy with your vegan shift.

No Need to Ditch your Favorite Restaurants

As veganism is becoming more popular, vegan options are also increasingly being included in nearly every restaurant's menu. Even if your food choice at a restaurant seems vegan, you still should inform your waiter about your dietary needs to ensure that no animal products are used in preparing the meal. For instance, a seemingly vegan meal may be made with chicken stock or butter.

Being Vegan Doesn't Have to Be Expensive

Meat, at more or less $3 per pound, is one of the grocery store's most expensive items, thus, you can easily save more if you purchase more produce. You can also save more by switching some of your fresh produce items for frozen ones.

Calcium from Plants

The National Institutes of Health recommends that adults, from ages 19 to 50, get at least 1,000 mg of calcium daily. However, preliminary findings indicate that vegans can still benefit with less than that amount.

In a European Journal study, when vegans consumed 525 mg of calcium a day, their risk of bone fracture was the same as those of meat eaters with a similar calcium intake. It's important to eat various naturally calcium-rich foods like kale, almonds, soybeans, bok choy, navel orangesand figs. For vegans, it's also important to consume foods fortified with calcium like plant-based milks, cereals and tofu with calcium sulfate.

Plus, leafy greens, fortified foods and soy are high in Vitamin C, which aids in calcium absorption.

Chapter 5 - Healthy Eating as a Vegan

A vegan diet is devoid of all animal products including milk, protein, yogurt, eggs, cheese and meat. It also excludes foods made with animal by-products like gelatin and food color. Whole grains, legumes, beans, nuts, fruits and vegetables make up the bulk of vegan diets.

What a healthful and delicious existence it is to switch to the vegan diet. But just because you can no longer eat or use animal products does not mean that your diet should be riddled with poor food choices that are void of natural nutrients. Thus, you need to be mindful of substances like artificial sweeteners, sugar, processed food items and white flour, all of which may harm your health in the long run.

The Importance of Protein

If you are new to veganism, you may wonder if you are getting adequate protein in your diet. As animal sources are rich in protein, you don't really need to eat steaks or burgers to experience a nutritious and healthy vegan protein diet. When you remove animal products from your diet, you need to be creative when it comes to your food selection in order to take in healthy protein levels.

When your protein intake is not enough, the body will use up muscle for fuel, leading to sluggish metabolism and a slight increase in body fat. A common vegan diet misconception is that it is difficult to consume adequate protein. However, you can easily obtain more than enough protein from your vegan diet.

Complete proteins are mainly found in animal products and their protein contains 20 amino acids required by the body. Mostly found in vegetables, fruits, nuts and beans, incomplete proteins contain some of the 20 amino acids. Thus, the amino acids not present in certain foods should be derived from other foods, so you can enjoy a diet that satisfies your daily protein requirement.

Below are some tips to help you get complete protein in your vegan diet:

Regularly add soy products into your diet. Soy is a source of complete protein.

Increase your intake of nuts and legumes as such foods have the most protein content available in smaller servings.

Eat various foods like nuts, seeds, legumes, vegetables, fruits and whole grains.

Meal Planning

There are no fixed rules to dictate the transition to a vegan diet. However, it may help if you adhere to a diet similar to the one that you have been consuming—just without the junk. Following a vegan diet doesn't mean your food choices will radically change. It just means that you will substitute some of the foods you are eating.

For example, you may still eat burritos. Instead of the cheese and meat, you may put in vegan cheese, salsa, beans, and vegan meat to your burrito. Psychological roadblocks, like being used to a particular diet for quite a while then making a sudden transition, can cause some people to fall off the bandwagon.

Looking for ways to consume 'transitional' foods will help maintain your resolve and go on with your vegan diet. If you love hamburgers, make a veggie burger and eat it with a side salad. If you love pizza, make it with loads of vegetables and vegan cheese. Prepare and eat vegan nuggets, instead of chicken nuggets.

Make stuffed peppers using a sautéed vegetables and seasoned rice and beans. Top with vegan cheese, bake, and enjoy. A baked potato with your favorite veggies, spices and vegan cheese always hits the spot. A homemade green juice or smoothie for breakfast, lunch, or dinner is a great source of liquid vitamins. Craving some dessert? You can eat baked apples drizzled with agave and cinnamon. You can also have pineapple chunks and dates. Or check the frozen section at your local natural foods store for a wide array of vegan ice creams. The choices for your vegan diet are truly endless.

The 30-Day Vegan Challenge

If you're new to veganism, challenge yourself to try it for 30 days. You can choose any day to start the vegan lifestyle. If you want what's best for your health and the environment, it's best to start this new lifestyle sooner rather than later. Here are some tips to make it easier:

1) Eliminate animal products from your refrigerator and your pantry. These include animal-based fats (butter, anyone?), eggs, dairy and meat. Also, you need to eliminate canned or boxed items that contain animal byproducts. Do this all at once.

2) Purchase a vegan cookbook. If you want to save money, you can get recipes online that contain a multitude of delicious and nutritious vegan recipes.

3) For your first month, craft a meal plan to include breakfast, lunch, and dinner. You should also include snacks.

4) With your new meal plan, make your grocery list.

5) Aside from shopping at your usual grocer, you should also shop at the nearest Whole Foods or local health food store.

At the end of the 30 day challenge, you may find out that you don't have to be dependent on your meal planning, recipes and cookbooks. By that time, you may have become an experienced vegan chef and shopper.

You may also notice that you are lighter by a few pounds. You may be more energetic and you may have to explain to friends the 'new glow' on your face.

Going vegan is a learning curve. To live a vegan lifestyle in a non-vegan world takes both curiosity and courage. Veganism is still a relatively new concept, even though it has been around for more than 70 years. You should allow yourself time to know more about veganism's various strands. And remember to congratulate yourself on your progress.

Moreover, if you have faith in yourself, a vegan lifestyle may soon become second nature to you. Remind yourself of the reasons why you are going vegan, and remember its benefits. When you go vegan, you are benefiting the environment, the animal kingdom, and the entire human population.

Chapter 6 - Other Vegan Living Aspects

Being vegan is not only about eating healthy and nutritious plant-based foods. It also encompasses other aspects of life, including entertainment, medical charities and medicine, among others.

Entertainment

Vegans do not support any kind of animal exploitation. Therefore, vegans avoid visiting aquariums and zoos. They also don't go to horse or dog-racing events. Instead, vegans would rather visit and support animal sanctuaries that provide loving and safe homes for rescued or abandoned animals.

Medical Charities

If you support a medical charity, you may want to know whether your chosen charity conducts animal testing. There are numerous charities that don't do animal tests and a lot of vegans seek to donate to charitable organizations that seek alternative testing methods.

Medicine

Most modern medicines are tested on animals before they are considered safe for human use. Vegans should also ask your pharmacist or your doctor about this, and also ask them to provide you with medication free of animal by-products like lactose or gelatin.

The Benefits of Veganism

Deciding to shift to a vegan diet and lifestyle is a choice that will lead to awesome health benefits as a result of the emphasis on nutritious, whole foods.

Studies indicate that vegans enjoy more health benefits as compared to individuals eating diets that are junk food and meat-heavy.

A vegan diet, with the appropriate food combinations to ensure the ingestion of B vitamins and amino acids, reduces heart disease risk, diabetes risk, and cancer risk. A vegan diet also can improve or eliminate symptoms in people suffering from inflammatory conditions.

Conclusion

Thank you again for downloading this book!

I hope this book was able to each you more about veganism, the principles behind it, and how to seamlessly switch to the vegan lifestyle. And above all I hope it inspires you to join the movement of vegans rising.

Together, we can make a difference for ourselves, for others, for animals, and for the planet.

Thank you and good luck!

Part 2

Introduction

Congratulations on downloading this book. Thank you for doing so. The following chapters will discuss many different foods and methods to prepare them using the Vegan way of eating.

Throughout the book, you will notice some of the recipes will have 'divided' mentioned in the recipe's ingredient listing. In case you didn't know, divided means the component will be used in more than one instance. For example, you may see a recipe written with 2 cups, divided. That could mean you will be using ½ of a cup in one part and 1 ½ cups in another segment of the recipe. Simple abbreviations will include 'c' fir cup, 't' for teaspoon, 'tbsp.' for tablespoon, EVOO for extra-virgin olive oil, and others.

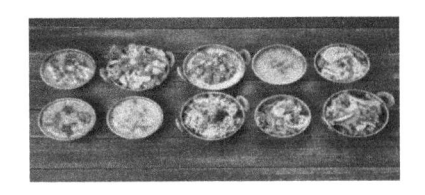

By following the Vegan lifestyle, you can help prevent diseases such as these:

- Arthritis
- Cardiovascular disease
- Blood pressure issues
- Type 2 Diabetes
- Osteoporosis
- Several forms of cancer

And many others.

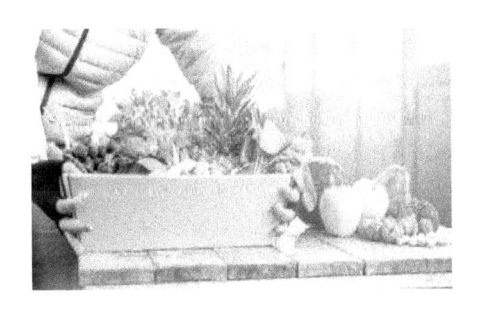

Not to mention, you can gain so many nutritional benefits from vegetables, fresh fruits, nuts, beans, whole grains, and soy products. These are some of those benefits and how your health can be affected:

- **Antioxidants**
  With this addition, you can protect your body against various types of cancer.
- **Carbohydrates**
  Your body burns your muscle tissue if you don't eat plenty of carbs.
- **Vitamin** C
  The C vitamin works as an antioxidant and helps keep your gums healthy. Your bruises will also heal faster.
- **Protein**
  As a vegan, lentils, nuts, peas, beans, and soy products provide this resource without the health issues that are associated with red meats.

- **Potassium**
  Acidity and water are balanced by potassium which also leads to a

reduction in cancer and cardiovascular diseases.
- **Fiber**

   The vegans experience better bowel movements with the increased high fiber in veggies and fruits.
- **Reduced saturated fats**

   Without the meats and dairy products, these levels are reduced immensely.
- **Magnesium**

   With the assistance of magnesium, calcium is better absorbed. It is found in dark leafy greens, seeds, and nuts.

There is a multitude of books on this subject on the market, so thanks again for choosing this one! You will soon discover how simple it is to maintain a healthy vegan diet and still enjoy your food. Using a slow cooker or crockpot, the stovetop, microwave, oven, and other kitchen appliances, you will learn how easy it is to have a tasty treat or dessert any time you choose.

Every effort was made to ensure that, as much as possible, your new vegan cookbook is full useful information with the serving amounts and times provided. Each of the recipes has a step-by-step process which is fully explained. Please enjoy!

Chapter 1: Breakfast Choices

Whether you decide to have a glass, cup, or bowl. Here are some delicious ways to begin your day.

Beverages

Apple Pear Cider in the Slow Cooker

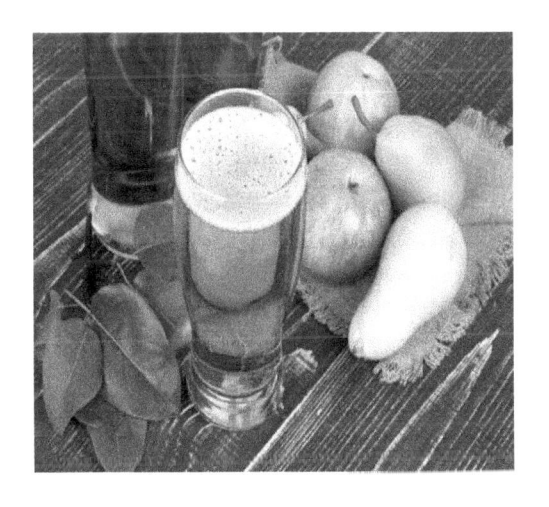

Makes: 12 cups

Total preparation time: 5 hrs. 18 min.

Ingredients:
- 1 orange, not peeled
- 2 pears
- 7 medium apples
- 4 t. of ground nutmeg
- 3 cinnamon sticks
- ½ t. of ground cloves
- ½-1 cup sweetener of your choice
- 12 c. of water

Directions:
1. Wash and slice all of the fruits, set the peelings and seeds to the side.
2. Add the spices, half of the sweetener, and water. Close the cooker lid.
3. Cook for 4 hours. Remove the lid and mash the fruit with a potato masher. Put the top back on, and let it simmer for 1 hour.
4. When it's ready to serve, add more sweetener if desired. Strain the fruit pulp through a mesh strainer.
5. Enjoy and serve anytime. It's also good cold!

Dirty Chai

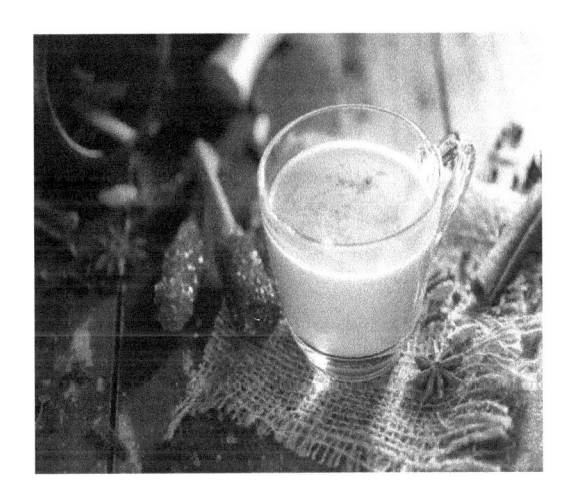

Makes: 2 servings

Total preparation time: 3 hrs. 10 min.

Ingredients:
- ½ c. of freshly-brewed coffee or espresso
- 1 ¼ c. of non-dairy milk
- 2 star anise
- 2 large orange peels
- 1 cinnamon stick

- 6 drops of stevia liquid, vanilla and/or any additional sweetener of your choice
- 4 white or black peppercorns

Need: 1.5-quart slow cooker

Directions:
1. Add all of the ingredients into the slow cooker and set the heat on low. Cook for three to four hours on low or cook it on high for two to three hours.
2. Strain and discard the solids. Serve and enjoy!

Iced Thai Tea Concentrate

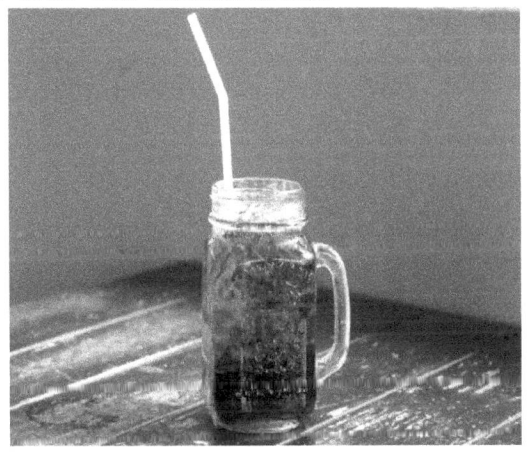

Makes: 6 Cups

Total preparation time: 4 hrs. 5 min. (Low setting)

Ingredients:
- 6 c. of water
- 4 whole cloves
- 2 whole cinnamon sticks
- 4 whole star anise
- 1 t. of cardamom seeds
- 8 tea bags, green or black loose tea (8-10 tbsp.) in a large tea bag
- 2 t. of orange flower water

- 1 t. of vanilla extract
- ½ c. of one of these:
- Maple syrup
- Stevia
- Coconut sugar, unsweetened

Optional: 1 small, quartered red beet

*Directions***:**
1. Pour the water into the slow cooker along with the spices (in a spice bag) and the beets. Cook for 4 hours on low heat.
2. After the 4 hours are over, remove the beets and spice bag.
3. Add the tea bags and turn up the heat to high. Boil for 5 minutes.
4. Dispose of the tea bags. Add your sweetener of choice, vanilla, and orange flower water.
5. Use approximately, ½ non-dairy milk, & ½ concentrate.
6. Serve and enjoy.

Other Breakfast Dishes

Blueberry Banana Muffins

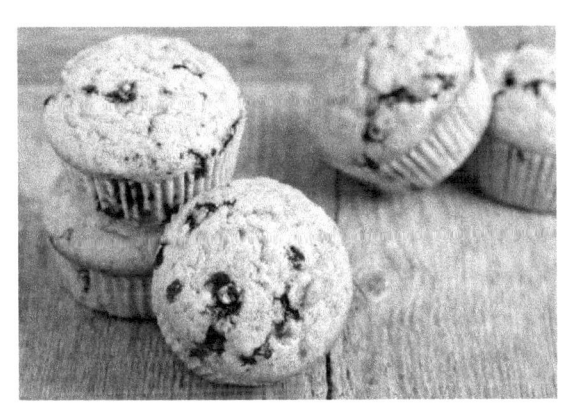

Makes: 12 servings

Total preparation time: 30 mins.

Ingredients:
- ½ c. beet sugar or other approved vegan substitute for sugar
- 2 overripe mashed bananas
- ½ t. of each:
- Salt
- Baking powder
- ¾ c. of all-purpose flour

- 1 ½ tbsp. of dry egg substitute
- ½ c. of whole wheat pastry flour
- 2 tbsp. of water
- ½ c. of blueberries

Also needed: Muffin tin
Optional: Paper muffin liners

Directions:
1. Set the oven's temperature to 350ºF.
2. Lightly grease the tins with some cooking spray or paper liners.
3. Combine the two kinds of flour, baking powder, salt, sugar, and mashed bananas in a mixing container until it's creamy.
4. In another dish, mix the water and egg replacement.
5. Stir all of the ingredients together then add the berries.
6. Add about ¼ cup of the batter to each of the cups.
7. Bake until it's golden (approx. 20-25 min.).

Crepes

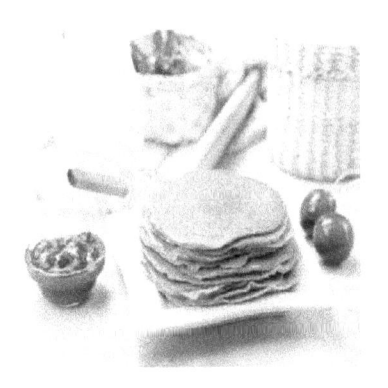

Makes: 4 servings

Total preparation time: 2 hrs. 25 min

Ingredients:
- ½ c. of each:
- Water
- Soy milk
- ¼ c. of melted soy margarine
- 2 t. of maple syrup
- 1 t. of turbinado sugar
- 1 c. of unbleached all-purpose flour
- ¼ t. of salt

Directions:

1. In a large container, mix all of the ingredients. Cover and chill for two hours.
2. Grease a skillet lightly with some margarine and warm it up until it's hot enough.
3. Empty the batter by three tablespoons into the pan. Cook until browned and flip. Serve.

Pancakes with Bananas

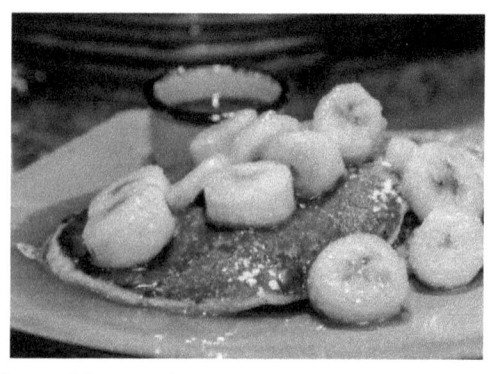

Makes: 12 servings

Total preparation time: 35 min.

Ingredients:

- 2 t. of baking powder
- ¾ c. of each:
- Whole wheat pastry flour
- Unbleached all-purpose flour
- 1 t. of egg substitute
- Dash of salt
- 1 c. of each:
- Rice or soy milk
- Ripe bananas, mashed (2-3 pieces)
- 1 t. of each:
- Fresh lemon juice
- Applesauce/Lighter Bake/Prune Puree
- ¼ c. of warm water

Optional: 1/3 c. of fresh blueberries

Directions:
1. Combine the two flours, baking powder, and salt.
2. In a separate dish, whisk the egg substitute and water until it becomes bubbly.
3. Blend in the water, soy/rice milk, lighter bake/applesauce, and bananas.

4. Mix in the liquid with the dry ingredients until they're barely incorporated. Blend in the berries.
5. Spoon the batter onto a griddle (medium heat). Add ¼ cup for each pancake. When the cakes start to bubble, flip, and cook until browned.
6. Transfer to a serving dish and enjoy.

Pancakes with Sweet Potatoes

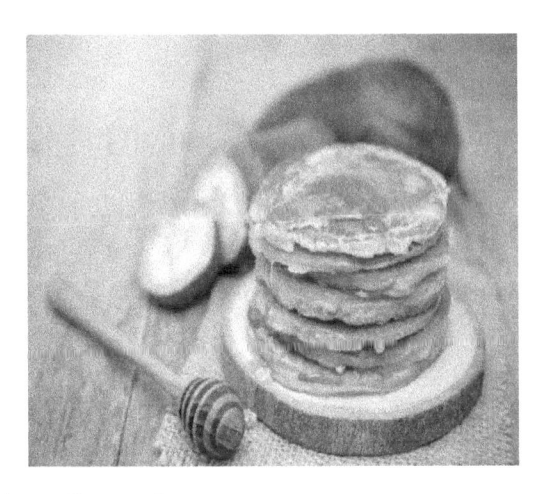

Makes: 3 servings

Total preparation time: 20 min.

Ingredients:
- 1 t. of ground cinnamon/allspice
- ½ t. of salt
- 1 ½ c. of whole wheat flour
- 1 c. of nondairy milk
- 3 t. of baking powder
- 3 t. of coconut sugar
- ¼ t. of baking soda
- 3 t. of vegan butter

- 1/3 c. of cooked sweet potato/yam
- ¼ c. of water
- 1 t. of each:
- Vanilla extract
- Apple cider vinegar or lemon juice

Optional: Cooking oil

Ingredients (Caramel Sauce):

- ½ c. coconut sugar
- ½ t. salt
- 2 t. of each:
- Cashew butter
- Water
- ½ c. of packed yam or sweet potato
- ¼ c. of non-dairy milk
- ¼ t. of allspice or ground cinnamon

*Directions***:**

1. Blend in the cinnamon, salt, flour, coconut sugar, baking powder, and baking soda. Pour the water, milk, vanilla, vinegar, butter, potato, and flax into a blender. Mix until it becomes smooth.

2. Combine the wet and dry ingredients. Don't use the blender. After mixing, let it rest for five to ten minutes.
3. Prepare a pan or griddle and warm it over medium heat (375ºF).
4. Prepare the sauce in a saucepan. Add the water and sugar. Remove from the burner.
5. Rinse out the mixer, and add ¼ cup of milk, cashew butter, potato, cinnamon, and salt. Mix all the ingredients well and add more milk if you want a different consistency. Transfer back to the burner and heat.
6. Pour the batter into the griddle and cook for 5 min. Flip the pancakes and finish cooking, this should take 4 min.
7. Serve and enjoy with the sauce. You can also add some chopped pecans or walnuts.

Quinoa & Strawberry Infused Cereal

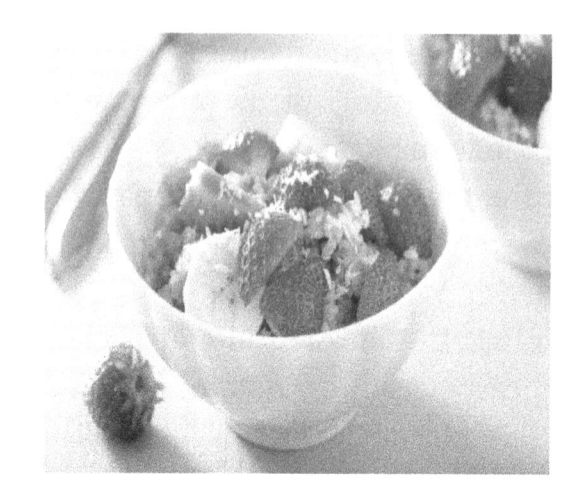

Makes: 1 serving

Total preparation time: 5 min.

Ingredients:
- 1 c. of strawberries, frozen
- 1 packet of stevia or 1 t. of liquid sweetener
- ¾ c. of water
- ¼ c. of cashews
- 1 c. of cooked quinoa

Toppings:
- Almonds

- Goji berries
- Blueberries

Directions:
1. Use a high-powered blender to combine the berries, water, cashews, and sweetener.
2. Add the prepared quinoa into the bowl, add milk, and drizzle with your preferred toppings.

Scrambled Tofu

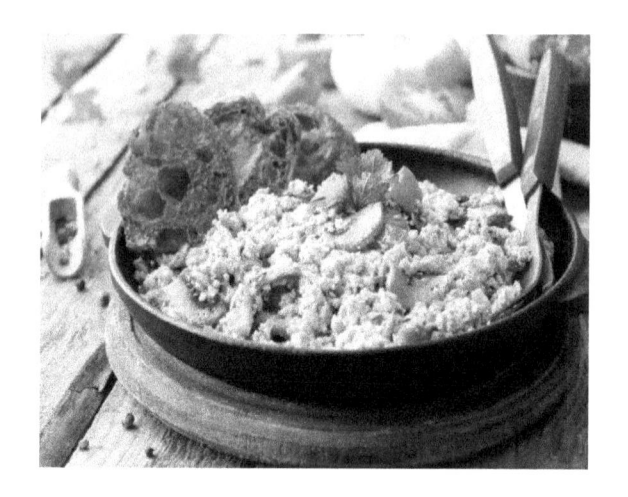

Makes: 4 servings

Total preparation time: 25 min.

Ingredients:
- 1 bunch of chopped green onions
- 1 tbsp. of olive oil
- 1 can of diced tomatoes (14 ½ oz.)
- 1 pkg. (12 oz.) of firm silken tofu
- Pepper and salt
- Ground turmeric

Optional: ½ c. vegan cheese

Directions:
1. Chop and sauté the onions. Over medium heat, heat up oil in a skillet, and slowly cook the onions until they're translucent.
2. Blend in the tomatoes along with the juices and the mashed tofu.
3. Add the turmeric, pepper, and salt for flavoring and lower the heat.
4. Garnish as desired.

Veggie Omelet in the Crock Pot

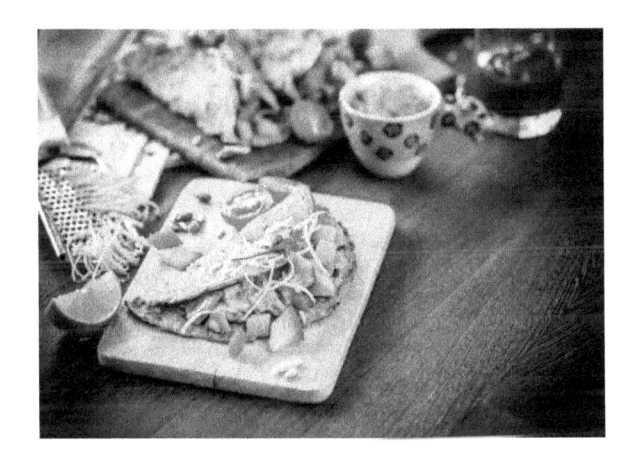

Makes: 4 servings

Total preparation time: 2 hrs. 10 min.

Ingredients:
- ½ c. of milk
- 6 eggs
- Pepper to taste
- 1/8 tsp. of each:
- Chili powder
- Garlic powder
- 1 small onion
- 1 red bell pepper
- 1 c. of broccoli florets
- 1 clove of garlic

Also needed:
- Electric mixer
- Non-stick cooking spray

Garnish:
- Chopped tomatoes and onions
- Shredded cheddar cheese
- Fresh parsley

Directions:

1. Lightly spray the crockpot. Finely chop the onions, mince the garlic, and cut the pepper into thin slices.
2. Blend the garlic powder, chili powder, pepper, salt, milk, and eggs in a large mixing container. Mix until well they're combined.
3. Toss in the garlic, onions, peppers, and florets to the cooker. Slowly mix in the egg mixture.
4. Secure the top on the crockpot and cook for 2 hours over high heat. Check it after 1 ½ hours. If the eggs are set, then that means the omelets are done.
5. Sprinkle the cheese and wait for 2-3 minutes. Turn off the cooker and slice the omelet into eight wedges.
6. Arrange on a serving platter and garnish with some chopped onions and tomatoes. Top it off with some fresh parsley.

Chapter 2: Lunchtime Favorites

Butternut Squash & Macaroni in the Crock Pot

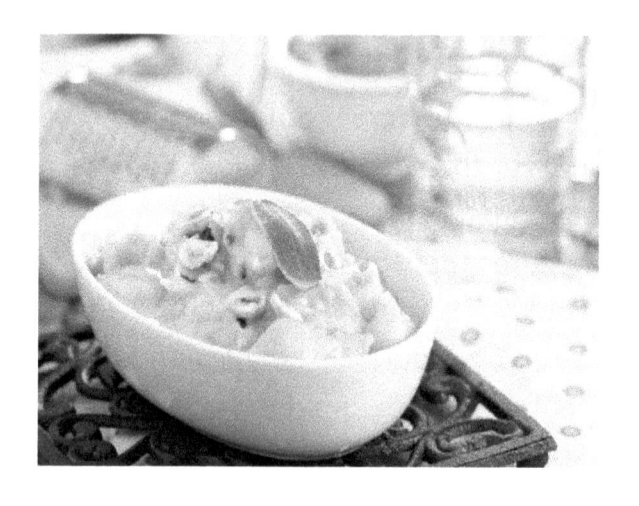

Makes: 5 cups

Total preparation time: 8 hrs. 15 min.

Ingredients (Morning):
- 1 ½ c. of each:
- Butternut squash

- Water
- ½ c. of chopped tomatoes
- 2 minced cloves of garlic
- 3 (3-in.) sprigs of thyme
- 1 (2-in.) fresh rosemary sprig

Ingredients (Evening):
- ½-1 c. of unsweetened non-dairy milk
- ¼ c. of nutritional yeast flakes
- 1 ½ c. of uncooked whole wheat macaroni
- Pepper and salt to taste

Needed: 1 ½-2 quart slow cooker

Directions:
1. Mix the morning ingredients and leave it for seven to nine hours on low heat.
2. Approximately 45 minutes before eating, purée the contents of the cooker using a blender along with the yeast and non-dairy milk. Add it back to the crockpot. Set the heat to high.
3. Mix in the macaroni and cook it covered for 20 minutes.

4. If it's too thick, add a little water and cook until the pasta is done. Flavor with some pepper and salt.

Note: Check the pasta every ten minutes until you are sure how fast your cooker can prepare the pasta.

Cauliflower Alfredo with Parmesan

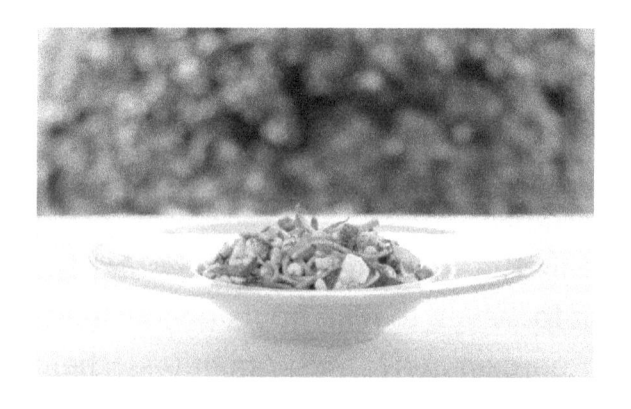

Makes: 6 servings
Total preparation time: 20 min.

Ingredients:
- 4 c. of cauliflower florets
- ¼ c. of silken or softened tofu
- 1 ½ c. of unsweetened almond or soy milk
- ½ c. of lemon
- 2 t. of Dijon mustard
- 1 ½ t. of each:
- Sea salt
- Onion powder
- ¼ t. of black pepper or more for the garnish
- 1 t. of garlic powder
- 1 lb. of your favorite pasta, cooked

Garnish (Optional):
- Vegan parmesan
- Freshly chopped parsley

Directions:
1. Chop the cauliflower into bite-sized pieces and steam them for 10-12 minutes. Toss the cauliflower pieces into a blender after steaming.

2. Pour in the lemon juice, milk, mustard, tofu, salt, onion powder, pepper, and garlic powder. Blend for 1-2 minutes until it's perfectly smooth.
3. Combine all of the ingredients and toss.
4. Serve with your favorite toppings such as parmesan, parsley, or more pepper.

'Jazz it up' and bring in the variety
- **Chicken & Broccoli Alfredo**
- Combine the sauce with vegan-grilled chicken strips and some steamed broccoli.

- **White Sauce Pizza**
- Purchase your favorite 'store-bought' pizza dough or whole-wheat pita. Top it off with the diced red bell pepper, corn, broccoli, and a drizzle of cheese sauce. You can also use 'store-bought' vegan mozzarella shreds for a simpler item.
- Bake for 15 minutes at 350ºF. Yummy!

Corn Risotto in the Slow Cooker

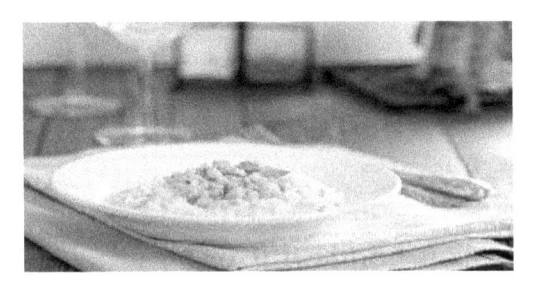

Makes: 3 cups

Total preparation time: 1 hr.

Ingredients:
- ½ c. of each:
- Arborio rice
- Kernel corn or 1 medium cob cut into four pieces
- 2 c. of water
- 2 t. of chopped fresh basil
- 3 (2-in.) thyme sprigs
- Salt and pepper to taste

Garnish: Additional chopped basil

Needed: 1 ½ to 2-quart slow cooker

Directions:
1. Combine the rice, water, and corn in the cooker. Add the four cob pieces (yes, the cob and all) along with the thyme to the mixture.
2. Cook for one hour or up to one and one-half hours. If it is dry after cooking for 45 minutes, just add a little water.
3. Remove the thyme stems and cob segments. Mix in the basil and serve.

Curried Carrot Fritters

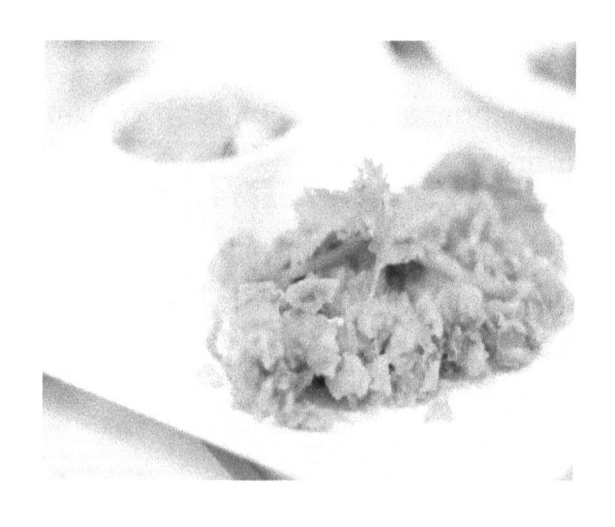

Makes: 7 fritters

Total preparation time: 22 min.

Ingredients:
- 1 med. onion
- 3 large carrots
- 2 finely chopped garlic cloves
- 2 t. of curry powder
- ¾ tbsp. of salt
- 1 c. of chickpea flour or *besan* flour
- ¼ t. of each:
- Ground ginger
- Ground coriander
- 1 t. of ground flax seed
- ½ c. of fresh cilantro or parsley
- ½ t. each of:
- Chili flakes (Optional)
- Fennel seed
- Cumin seeds
- ¼ c. of water

Needed: Food processor

Directions:

1. Grate the carrot and onion. The processor attachment is great for this.
2. Combine the garlic, onions, and carrots in a large container and mix well. Add the remainder of the ingredients (don't include the water yet) and mix well. Now, pour in the water and stir. The batter will be thick. Let it rest for ten minutes or so.
3. Set the oven's temperature to 400ºF.
4. Use a *Silpat* or parchment paper to line a baking tin. Arrange the dough in 1/3 cup portions and flatten (½-inch).
5. Cook for 20-25 minutes. Flip once after about 15 minutes.

Kale & Sweet Potato Hash

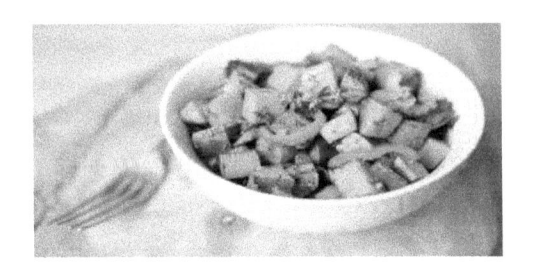

Makes: 4 servings

Total preparation time: 40 min.

Ingredients:
- 1 chopped onion
- 2 med. sweet potatoes
- 2 tbsp. of olive oil
- 2 minced cloves of garlic
- ½ c. of low-sodium vegetable broth
- ½ t. of sea salt
- 1 t. of each:
- Dried rosemary

- Smoked paprika
- ¼ t. of ground black pepper
- 1 large bunch or 4 c. of curly kale

Directions:
1. Peel and chop the potatoes into ½-inch cubes. Prepare and measure the rest of the fixings.
2. Warm up the oil in a skillet over medium heat on the stovetop. Once it's hot, toss in the onions and sauté for 3 min. Add the garlic and cook until it's fragrant, can take a minute.
3. Stir in the potatoes, rosemary, and paprika. Sauté for 5 minutes and slowly pour in the broth. Place a lid on the pot and cook on low heat for about 7 minutes until it becomes bubbly.
4. Toss in the kale and cover the pot, cook until the kale is wilted (2 min.).
5. Season with the pepper and salt, let it simmer uncovered for 5 more minutes.
6. Serve when the potatoes are tender.

Quinoa Tabbouleh

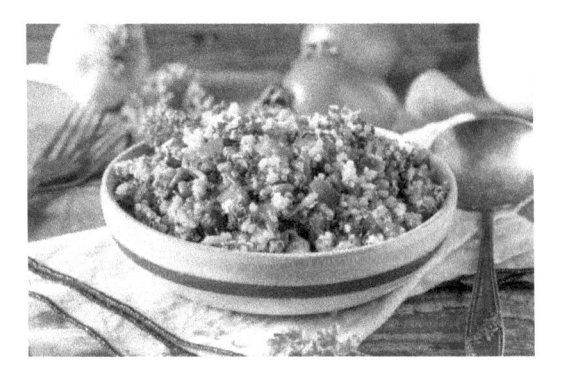

Makes: 6 servings

Total preparation time: 35 min.

Ingredients:
- 3 English cucumbers
- 4 c. of cooked & cooled quinoa
- 6 small tomatoes
- 1 large red onion
- 2 handfuls of chopped mint
- 6 handfuls parsley, chopped
- 1 t. of golden balsamic vinegar or apple cider vinegar
- Juice from 4 lemons
- ½ c. of olive oil
- Salt and pepper to taste

Directions:
1. Dice the veggies, and combine them with the quinoa, lemon juice, herbs, salt, pepper, and vinegar.
2. Pour the oil in ¼-cup increments until the quinoa is creamy and sticky.

Shepherd's Pie with Lentils

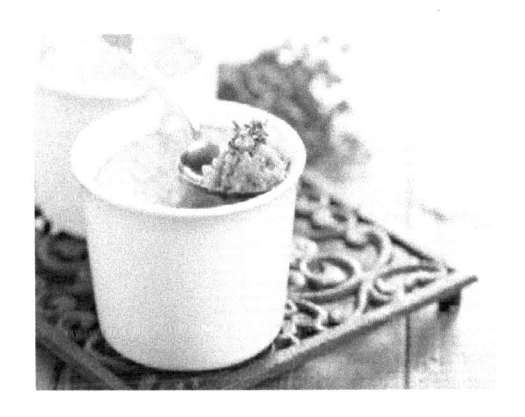

Makes: 6 servings

Total preparation time: 55 min.

Ingredients:
- 3 garlic cloves
- 1 large carrot
- 1 med. onion
- 3 t. of tamari
- 2 t. of cornstarch/arrowroot
- 2 ½ t. of dried herbs: rosemary, marjoram or thyme
- 1 c. of each:

- Vegetable or mushroom broth
- Crushed tomatoes or canned
- 2 ½ c. of cooked lentils
- 6 c. of raw potatoes
- 1/3 c. of unsweetened nondairy milk

Optional:
- 1 knob vegan butter
- Salt and Pepper

Directions:
1. Finely chop the garlic and onion. Dice the carrot and potatoes.
2. Prepare the oven in advance to 400ºF.
3. Boil the potatoes with a pinch of salt, simmering for approximately 15 minutes. Drain and add them back in the pan along with the butter and milk. Mash and set aside.
4. Heat up another skillet and cook the carrots, garlic, and onions until almost browned. Use a drop of water instead of oil if you wish.
5. Blend in the lentils, dried herbs, and cornstarch or arrowroot.

6. Then, mix in the tomatoes and tamari, along with the veggie broth, simmering until it starts to boil.
7. Empty the mixture into an oven dish and top with the mashed potatoes.
8. Arrange the pan on a cookie tin and bake for about 30 minutes.

Vegan Meatloaf with Gravy

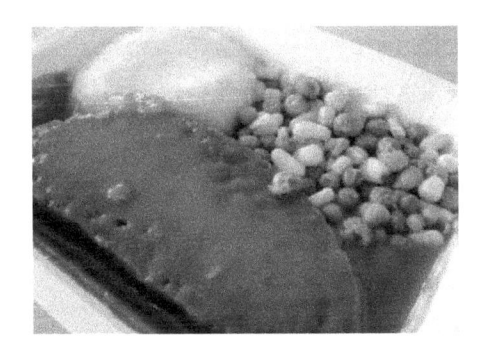

Makes: 8 thick slices

Total preparation time: 55 min.

Ingredients (Loaf):
- 2 large garlic cloves
- 1 small onion

- 1 c. of cooked:
- Red lentils
- Green lentils
- 3 c. of mushrooms
- ½ c. of each:
- Whole wheat/ spelt/rice/oat flour
- Walnut bits (for nut-free substitute: ½ c. oats or ½ c. sunflower seeds)

- ¼ c. of ground flax seeds
- 2 t. of dried thyme
- 1 t. of tamari
- 1 ½ t. of pepper and salt
- ½ c. of water

Ingredients (Gravy):
- 1 t. of each:
- Nutritional yeast
- Cornstarch/all-purpose flour/arrowroot
- 1 t. of tamari
- 2 chopped medium onions
- 2 c. of mushroom broth or 2 c. of water and 3 mushrooms

*Also need*ed:

- Parchment paper
- 2 (¾ x 8.5 x 4.5-in.) loaf pans

Directions (Loaf):

1. Use a food processor to chop the garlic, onions, and mushrooms until fine.
2. Set the oven temperature to 370ºF.
3. Blend all of the ingredients in a large mixing container but leave out the water. Using your hands, add just enough water for the mixture to combine.
4. Add a layer of paper in the tin to act as a handle for the finished loaf. Add the meatloaf and pack tightly.
5. Bake for 50 minutes, covering with a piece of aluminum foil if it starts to get too dark.
6. Let it cool for 15 minutes before serving.

Directions (Gravy):

1. Over low heat, sauté the onion and add it and the rest of the gravy ingredients in a mixer.
2. Blend until smooth. Pour into a pan over medium heat until hot.
3. Serve over the sliced loaf and enjoy.

Vegetable Curry

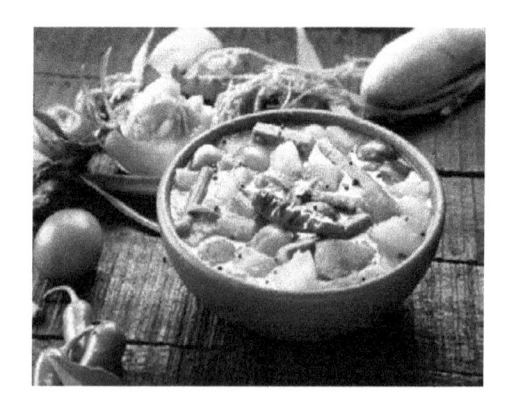

Makes: 6 servings

Total preparation time: 50 min.

Ingredients:
- 1 med. eggplant
- 3 garlic cloves

- 1 sweet potato
- 1 of each: green & red bell pepper
- 1 onion
- 2 carrots
- 6 t. of olive oil
- 1 t. of each ground:
- Turmeric
- Cinnamon
- ¾ t. of cayenne pepper
- 1 t. of curry powder
- ¾ tbsp. of sea salt
- ¼ c. of blanched almonds
- 1 can (15 oz.) of garbanzo beans
- 1 sliced zucchini
- 2 t. of raisins
- 10 oz. of spinach
- 1 c. of orange juice

Directions:
1. Chop or mince the veggies but slice the zucchini. Drain the beans.
2. Add the potato, peppers, eggplant, onion, carrots, and 3 tablespoons of the olive oil. Cook slowly for about five minutes over medium heat.

3. Add 3 tablespoons of the oil, turmeric, the garlic, pepper, salt, cinnamon, and curry powder. Continue cooking slowly for three more minutes.
4. Add the spice mixture with the beans, juice, raisins, zucchini, and almonds. Let it simmer, covered, for 20 minutes.
5. Lastly, add the spinach. Cook for five more minutes and serve.

Chapter 3: Healthy Soups & Stews

Soups

Butternut Squash Soup in the Slow Cooker

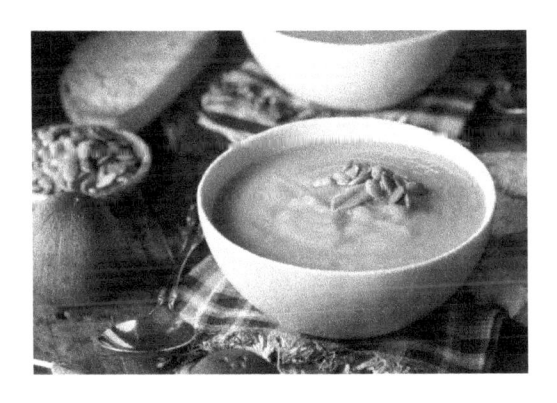

Makes: 8 servings

Total preparation time: 6 hrs. 20 min.

Ingredients:
- 1 lb. of butternut squash
- 1 med. diced onion
- 1 granny smith apple, peeled & sliced
- ½ lb. of carrots
- 3 c. of vegetable broth

- 1 t. each of salt and pepper
- 1 bay leaf
- ¼ t. of dried ground sage
- 1 can (13.5 oz.) of coconut milk

*Also need*ed: Immersion blender

Directions:

1. Peel and cube the apples, squash, and carrots. Toss into the cooker along with the onion, bay leaf, and broth. Secure the lid and cook six hours on the low setting. (The veggies should be softened.)
2. Discard the leaf and add the contents to the blender. Puree until creamy. Pour it back into the cooker along with the milk, sage, salt, and pepper.
3. Serve with some crusty bread or croutons.

Coconut Curry Chickpea Lentil Soup

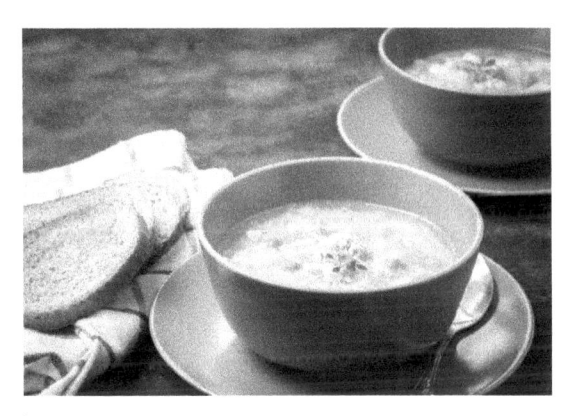

Makes: 7 servings

Total preparation time: 4 hrs. 10 min.

Ingredients:
- 1 c. of dry lentils
- 6 c. of vegetable broth
- 2 cans (15 oz. ea.) of garbanzos or chickpeas
- 1 can (15 oz.) of lite coconut milk
- 1 large sweet potato
- 1 t. of each:
- Ground ginger
- Ground turmeric
- ¼ t. of pepper

- 2 t. of curry powder
  - ½ t. of salt

Also needed: Slow Cooker

Directions:
1. Pick and rinse the lentils. Drain the chickpeas. Slice the potato into small chunks.
2. Add each of the ingredients into the slow cooker. Stir well.
3. Use the high heat setting for four hours.
4. Flavor with the pepper and salt if desired.

Corn and Red Pepper Chowder

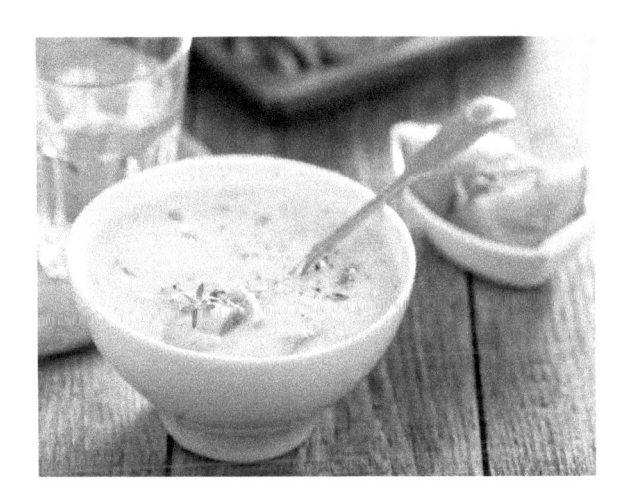

Makes: 4-6 servings

Total preparation time: 8 hrs. 30 min.

Ingredients:
- 2 tbsp. of olive oil
- 3 med. potatoes
- 1 med. red bell pepper
- 1 med. yellow onion
- 4 c. of each:

- Frozen sweet corn kernels, divided
- Vegetable broth
- 1 t. of each:
- Kosher salt
- Ground cumin
- 1/8 t. of cayenne pepper
- ½ t. of smoked paprika
- 1 c. almond or soy milk
- Black pepper and salt to taste

Ingredients (Garnish):

- Sliced scallions
- Corn kernels
- Red bell pepper

Also needed:

- Slow cooker
- Immersion blender

Directions:

1. Warm the oil on the stove top using medium heat. Toss in the onion and sauté approximately five minutes. Empty the onion into the cooker. Stir and add the potatoes, red pepper, 1 cup of the corn, salt, cayenne pepper, paprika, cumin, and the broth.

2. Set the timer for 4-6 hours on high or if you prefer 8-10 on the low setting.
3. When done, take off the lid, and let it slightly cool.
4. Purée the soup with the blender. Add the mixture to the cooker and turn it back on.
5. Stir in the milk and rest of the corn. Place a lid on the cooker and cook until hot (20-30 min.).
6. Serve and enjoy.

Homestyle Chickpea Noodle Soup

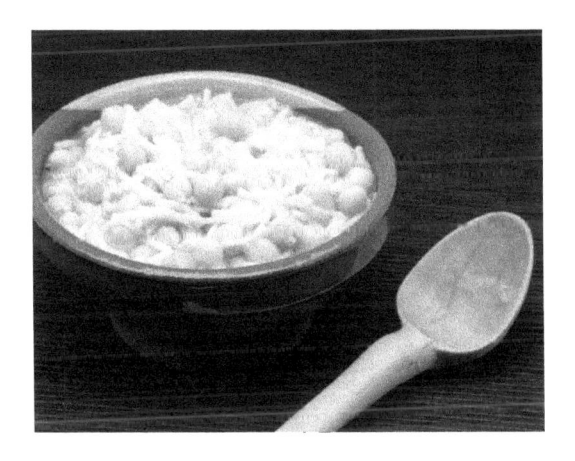

Makes: 6 servings

Total preparation time: 40 min.

Ingredients:
- 2 tbsp. of olive oil
- 4 garlic cloves, minced
- 4 celery stalks
- 2 med. onions
- 4 med. carrots
- 6-8 sprigs fresh thyme
- 2 quarts vegetable broth
- 1 bay leaf
- 8 oz. of whole wheat rotini noodles
- Salt and pepper to taste
- 1 c. of cooked chickpeas

*Garnish***:**
- Chopped fresh parsley
- Bread or crackers

*Directions***:**
1. Thinly slice the celery and carrots. Chop the onions.
2. Warm up the oil in a large pot. Using the medium heat setting, toss in the bay

leaf, fresh thyme, celery, carrots, onions, and garlic. Sauté the veggies until just softened.
3. Pour in the broth and let it boil. Empty the chickpeas and noodles into the mixture. Cook for eight minutes or until the noodles are done. Sprinkle with the pepper and salt if desired.
4. Take the pot off the burner and serve with your chosen garnishes.

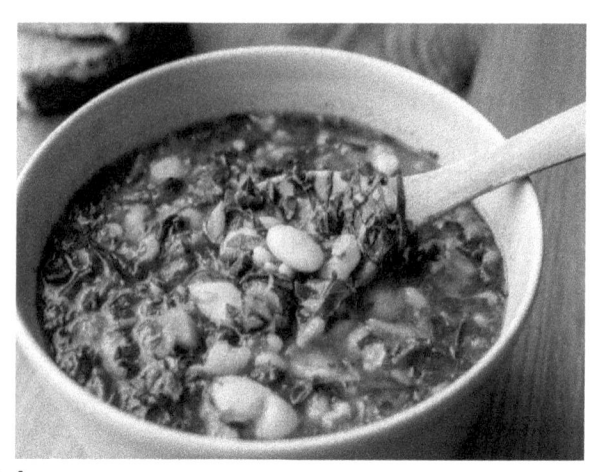

Kale soup

Makes: 8 servings

Total preparation time: 55 Minutes

Ingredients:
- 8 c. of water
- 1 chopped onion
- 2 t. of each:
- Chopped garlic
- Olive oil
- 1 bunch of kale
- 6 cubes of vegetable bouillon (Knorr)
- 1 can of diced tomatoes (15 oz.)
- 6 white potatoes

- 2 cans of cannellini beans (15 oz. each)
- 2 t. of dried parsley
- Salt and pepper to taste
- 1 t. of Italian seasoning

Directions:

1. Remove the stems from the kale and chop. Peel and cube the potatoes.
2. Use a large soup pot and pour in the oil along with the garlic and onion. Cook until softened.
3. Blend in the kale and cook about for two minutes until it's wilted.
4. Empty the water and the remainder of the ingredients. Simmer over medium heat for 25 minutes.
5. Sprinkle with salt and pepper to your liking.

Lentil and Apricot Soup in a Slow Cooker

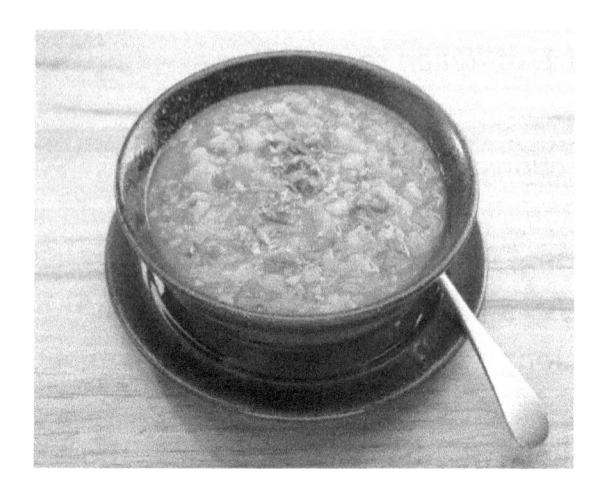

Makes: 4-6 servings

Total preparation time: 5 hrs. 5 min.

Ingredients:
- 1 diced onion
- 1 c. of red lentil
- 1 tbsp. of oil
- 1 diced clove of garlic
- 4 1/3 c. of water or stock
- ½ t. of turmeric
- 2 thin slices of fresh ginger

- 1 pinch of chili powder or flakes to taste
- 1 t. each of ground:
- Cumin seed
- Coriander seed
- ¼ c. dried apricot
- Pepper and salt
- Lemon salt or lemon juice as desired

Garnish: Chopped cilantro

Directions:
1. Prepare the lentils. Wash and drain.
2. Chop up the items that need to be chopped. Add all of the ingredients into the pot. Cook for 4-5 hours on low heat.
3. Garnish as desired and enjoy.

Stews & Chilis

Chickpea and Sweet Potato Chili

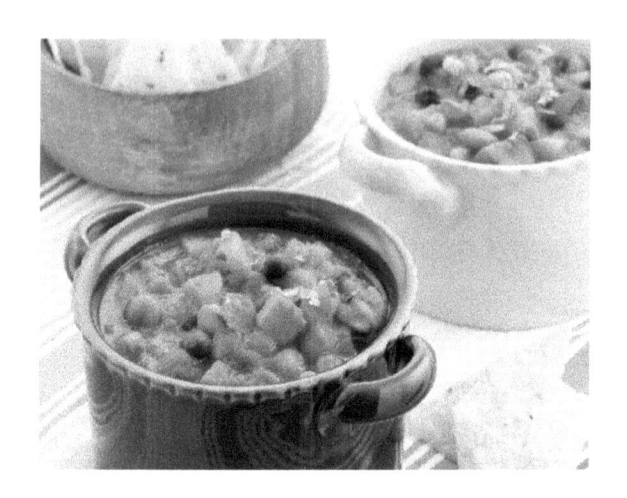

Makes: 8 servings

Total preparation time: 10 ½ hours

Ingredients:
- 1 large sweet potato
- 1 chopped chipotle pepper for spicy or 4 tbsp. adobo sauce (less spicy)
- 13.5 oz. canned tomato sauce
- 28 oz. canned diced tomatoes

- 2 cans (19 oz. each) chickpeas
- 2 carrots
- 2 medium onions
- 4 garlic cloves
- 2 t. chili powder
- ½ cup stock
- 1 t. of each:
- Salt
- Ground cumin
- Juice of ½ lime

Optional:
- Cilantro leaves
- Avocado
- Greek yogurt or sour cream
- Tortilla chips

Also needed: 5-quart slow cooker

Directions:
1. Peel and cut the potato into 1 ⅓ to 2-inch bits. Drain and rinse the chickpeas. Mince the carrots, onions, and mince the garlic.

2. Add all the ingredients to the cooker and stir until they're combined well. Place in the fridge until ready to cook.
3. Cook the ingredients for eight to ten hours on low heat.
4. Blend in the juice before serving.
5. Garnish as desired.

3-Bean Sweet Potato Chili

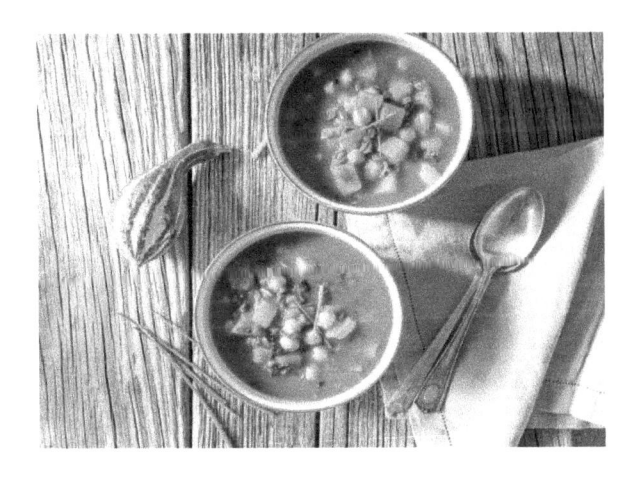

Makes: 8 servings

Total preparation time: 7 hrs. 10 min. -or less, depending on the method

Ingredients:
- 1 ½ c. of dried beans, soaked overnight
- 1 can (28 oz.) of crushed tomatoes
- 4 fat garlic cloves
- 1 large sweet potato
- 1 t. of mixed dried herbs

- 2 bay leaves
- ½ t. of smoked paprika
- 1-2 t. of dried chili flakes
- ¼ t. of each:
- Cacao, cocoa powder
- Ground cinnamon
- 1 t. of sugar
- 2 c. of water
- Pepper and salt

*Also need*ed**:** Slow Cooker

*Directions***:**
1. Peel and cube the onion and potato. You can use ½ cup of black-eyed peas, black beans, and lima beans for extra color and flavors.
2. Prepare the cooker for seven hours on low and four hours on high.
3. Otherwise, use a pan or the oven to mix all of the ingredients together well. Simmer the beans with a little oil, or not, in a pot or pan.

4. Cook for about three hours unless you use canned beans which would only need forty minutes.
5. If you chose the oven, cook at 300ºF and bake until tender.

Tomato-Curry Lentil Stew

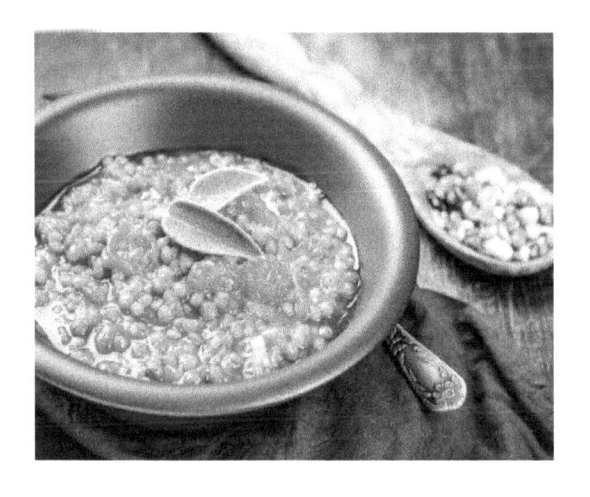

Makes: 2 servings

Total preparation time: 1 hr.

Ingredients:

- 1 c. of water
- ½ c. of dry lentils
- 5 oz. of stewed tomatoes
- 2 stalks of celery, leaves and chopped
- 1/8 c. of chopped onion
- ¼ t. of curry powder
- 3 minced garlic cloves
- Salt and pepper, to taste

Directions:
1. Add the water and lentils to a stew pot. When the lentils begin boiling, lower the heat setting to medium.
2. Toss in the celery, onion, and tomatoes. Put a lid on the pot and slowly cook for 45 minutes. Stir the mixture occasionally every 20 minutes. Pour in water as needed. For the last 15 minutes, add the spices.
3. Serve while piping hot!

Sides or veggies

Baked Spaghetti Squash

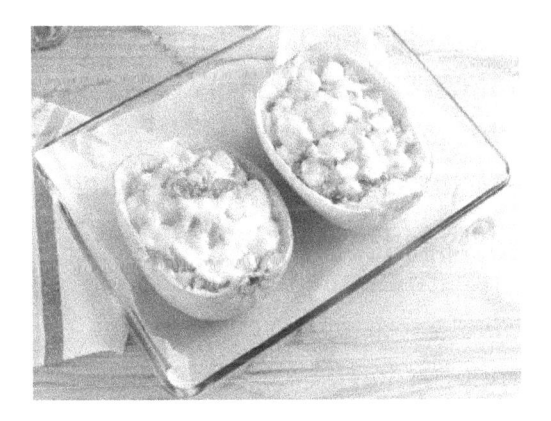

Makes: 6-8 servings

Total preparation time: 1 hr. 35 min.

Ingredients:

2 large spaghetti squash (3 -4 lbs. each)

Ingredients (Tofu Filling):
- 12 oz. of extra-firm tofu
- 3-4 tbsp. of EVOO

- 2 juiced lemons (1/3 c.)
- ½ t. of black pepper and sea salt to taste
- 3 t. of nutritional yeast
- 1 t. of dried oregano
- ¼ c. of vegan parmesan cheese, set aside an additional cup for serving
- ½ c. of packed fresh basil

Ingredients (Serving):

- 25 oz. red sauce or your favorite vegan marinara sauce
- Vegan parmesan cheese

Optional:

- Red pepper flakes
- Fresh chopped basil

Directions:

1. Line a large cookie sheet with foil and program the oven to 400ºF.
2. Drain and press the tofu for 10 minutes.
3. Cut the squash lengthwise with a sharp knife. Use a sharp spoon to remove the seeds and most of the stringy insides. Clean it out.

4. Coat the inside of the squash with the oil, salt, and pepper.
5. Place it with the cut-side down on the cookie sheet.
6. Bake for 45 minutes. When the knife easily cuts the flesh and skin, remove it from the oven and lower the heat to 375ºF.
7. Meanwhile, in a blender or food processor, mix all of the tofu ingredients, scraping the sides when needed. You want the texture to have bits of basil still in pieces.
8. Adjust the flavorings and add the nutritional yeast for the cheese flavoring and the lemon juice for a bit of tang.
9. When the squash is ready, use a fork to remove the fine strings of spaghetti. Set them to the side.
10. Grease a 9 x 13 (or something close). Place 1/3 of the squash followed by a few spoons of tofu ricotta, and a layer of sauce. Continue the process making the top layer sauce.

11. Cover the container with foil and bake for approximately 20 minutes. Take the foil off and bake for another 10 to 15 minutes. (If it is browning too quickly, cover it up with the foil.)
12. Let it cool or rest for a couple of minutes and enjoy.

Note: The dish will keep in the fridge for about two to three days. To reheat the meal, bake for 20-25 minutes in a 350 ºF.

BBQ Baked Beans

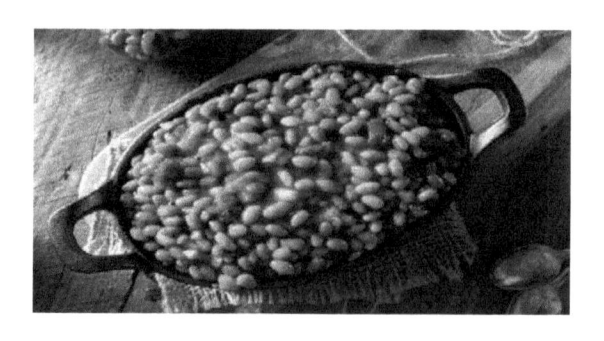

Makes: 8 servings

Total preparation time: 3 hrs. 55 min.

Ingredients:
- 1 ½ c. of small dried white beans or 4 ½ c. of canned beans
- 3 large garlic cloves
- 1 large onion
- 3 c. of (28 oz.) canned crushed tomatoes
- ½ c. of apple cider vinegar
- 1 heaping t. of wet mustard
- 1/3 c. of maple syrup
- 2 t. of blackstrap molasses
- 1 large bay leaf
- 1 t. of each:
- Dried rosemary
- Ground cumin
- Pepper
- ½ t. of chili powder or flakes
- 2 t. of salt
- 1 heaping t. of smoked paprika or liquid smoke, not both
- 1 c. of water

Directions:

1. Measure the beans before soaking overnight. Drain and add water until they simmer for 40 minutes. Drain and continue.
2. On the stove top, sauté the garlic and onions until they're transparent. Toss in the rest of the ingredients and continue cooking until it bubbles.
3. Lower the heat, place a lid on the pan, and cook about three hours. Stir often to make sure they don't stick.
4. In the oven, after the beans simmer, put them in a 300ºF oven for three to four hours until the beans are soft.

Tofu Noodles

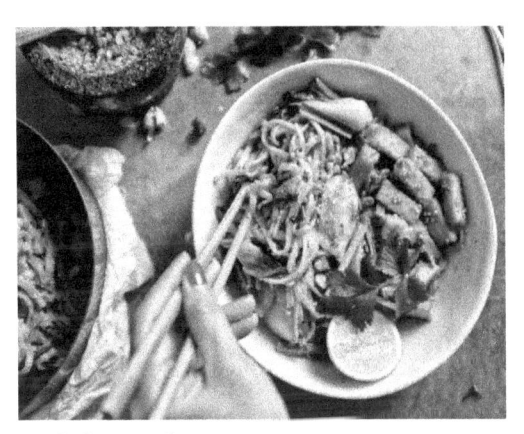

Makes: 6-8 servings

Total preparation time: 25-30 min.

Ingredients:
- 1 pkg. of vegan ribbon noodles, bow tie or shell pasta (8-10 oz.)
- 1 tbsp. of olive oil
- 1-1½ c. of brown or white mushrooms
- 3 celery stalks
- 1 mcd. onion
- 2 c. of unsweetened almond milk
- 3 tbsp. of unbleached white flour
- 1 pkg. (8 oz.) of baked tofu

- 1 c. of vegan mozzarella cheese (Optional)
- Salt and pepper to taste
- 2-3 scallions

Ingredients (Topping):
- Paprika
- Toasted breadcrumbs or wheat germ

Directions:
1. Finely chop the onions and tofu. Dice the celery stalks. Prepare the noodles until it's *al dente* then drain it.
2. Add the onion to a stir-fry pan and sauté until golden. Toss in the celery and sauté for another three to four minutes. Combine and sauté the mushrooms until wilted.
3. Add the flour, one tablespoon at a time, until it's well blended with the vegetables. Empty the milk, raising the heat, and cook until thickened.
4. Blend in the cheese, tofu, and scallions along with the noodles. Season with some pepper and salt.

5. Put a top on the pan and set aside for at least five minutes so the noodles can mix with the sauce.
6. Top off the dish with the crumbs or wheat germ and paprika.

Chapter 4: Delicious Sandwiches & Salads

Salads

Caesar Salad

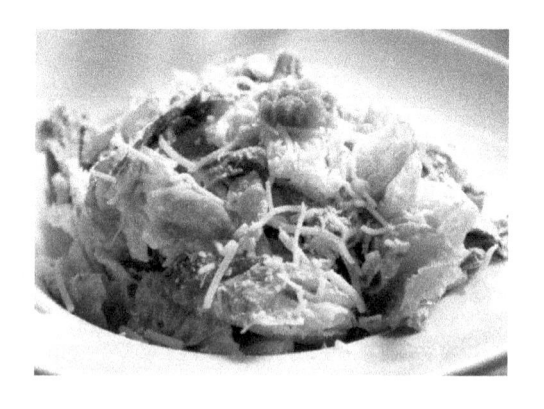

Makes: 4-6 servings

Total preparation time: 10 min.

Ingredients (Dressing):
- ½ c. of each:

Water
Walnuts

- 3 tbsp. of olive oil
- 1 t. of white miso paste
- Juice from ½ of a lime
- 1 t. of each:
- Dijon mustard
- Gluten-free tamari
- Garlic powder
- ½ t. of black pepper
- ¼ t. of sea salt

Ingredients (Salad):
- 1 c. cherry tomatoes, halved
- 2 heads of romaine lettuce, chopped
- Vegan parmesan 'store-bought' or Walnut Parmesan

Optional: Vegan croutons

Directions:
1. Prepare the dressing by combining all of the components in a blender. Mix well (for 2 min.) until it's slightly chunky which is more of a Caesar dressing texture.
2. Prepare the salad by tossing all of the ingredients with half of the prepared dressing.

3. Toss, adding as desired and serve.

Chickpea Tomatoes & Peppers Salad

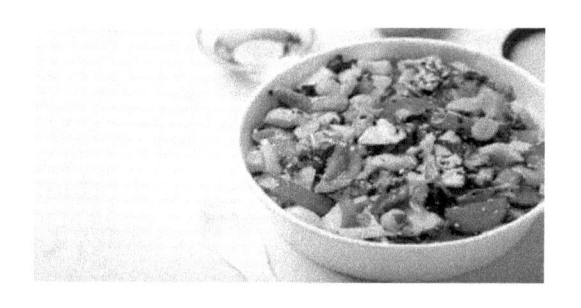

Makes: 4-6 servings

Total preparation time: 15 minutes

Ingredients:
- 3 med. ripened firm tomatoes
- 1 can of chickpeas (15-16 oz.)
- 1 jar of roasted red peppers (10-12 oz.)
- Juice from ½ a lemon

- Freshly sliced basil leaves
- 1 tbsp. of olive oil
- A pinch of salt & ground pepper

Optional:
- ½ c. of black olives
- Mixed baby arugula or greens

Directions:
1. Mix all of the components except for the greens. Combine well.
2. Serve with or without the greens.

Sauerkraut Salad

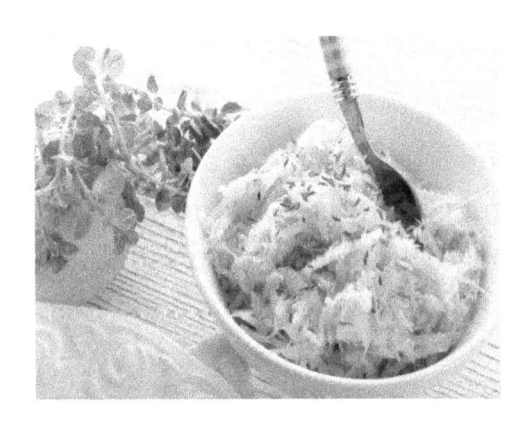

Makes: 6 servings

Total preparation time: 2 days 15 min.

Ingredients:
- 1 onion
- 2 celery stalks
- 1 quart drained sauerkraut
- 1 chopped of each:
- Large carrot
- Green pepper
- 1 jar (4 oz.) of drained pimento peppers
- 1 ½ c. of beet sugar
- 1 t. of mustard seed
- ½ c. of cider vinegar
- 1 c. of vegetable oil

Directions:
1. Chop the celery and onions and combine in a large mixing container along with the mustard seed, pimentos, carrots, green peppers, and sauerkraut.

2. Combine the vinegar, oil, and sugar in a saucepan. Cook until it boils then remove from the burner.
3. Empty the sugar mixture over the salad. Cover in the fridge for two days.

3-Bean Salad

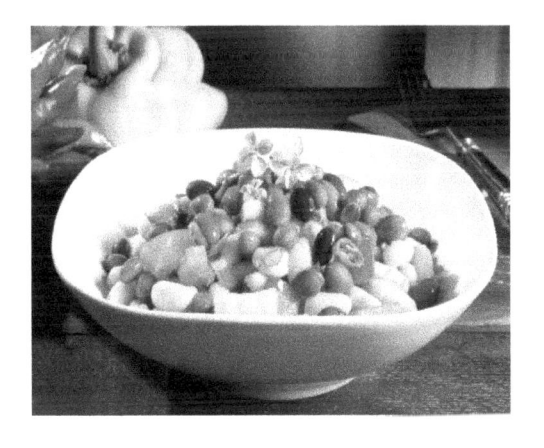

Makes: 8 servings

Total preparation time: 2 hrs. 15 min.

Ingredients:
- 1 can (15 oz.) of each:

- Green beans
- Kidney beans
- Garbanzo beans
- 1 stalk celery
- 4 green onions
- ½ c. of cider vinegar
- ¼ c. of vegetable oil
- ½ t. of ground dry mustard
- 1 tbsp. of honey
- ¼ t. of each:
- Ground black pepper
- Garlic powder

Optional:
- Onion powder
- Cayenne pepper

Directions:
1. Rinse and drain the beans and chop the onions and celery. Mix them in a bowl.
2. In another dish, whisk the remainder of the ingredients.
3. Empty the dressing over the salad and toss to combine.
4. Chill for about two hours.

Chapter 5: Dips, Snacks, & Appetizers

Dips & spreads

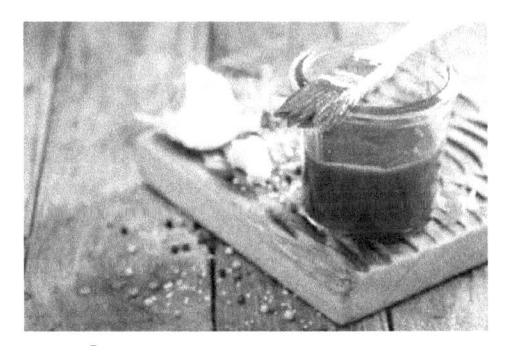

Barbecue Sauce

Makes: 2 ½ cups

Total preparation time: 1 hr.

Ingredients:
- 2 t. apple cider vinegar
- 15-16 oz. tomato sauce - 1 can
- 1 t. molasses or extra syrup
- 3 t. agave nectar or maple syrup

- 2-3 t. tamari or reduced-sodium soy sauce
- 1 t. of each:
- Basil or dried oregano
- Chili powder
- Smoked or sweet paprika

Directions:
1. Add all of the ingredients in a large container and whisk them together thoroughly.
2. Let it stand for one hour (if you have the time) for all of the tasty flavors to blend fully.

Black Olive Fig & Tapenade with Rosemary

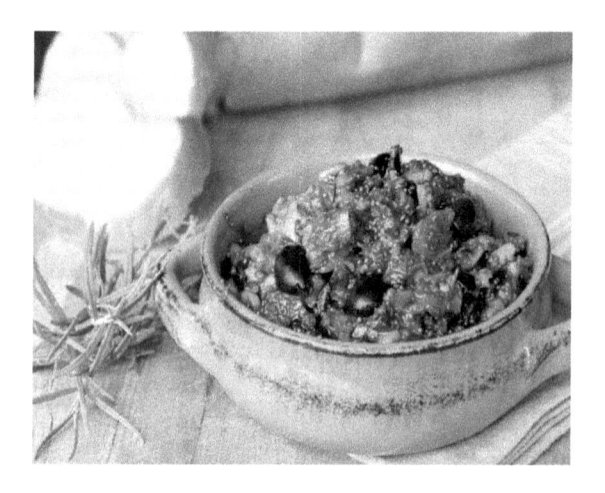

Makes: 1 Cup

Total preparation time: 25 min.

Ingredients:
- 6 fresh figs
- 1 jar or can (14 oz.) of black olives
- 1 garlic clove
- 2 tbsp. of EVOO (Extra Virgin Olive Oil)
- ½ t. of fresh rosemary

Directions:
1. For the fresh figs: Warm up the oven to 350ºF. Remove the stems and arrange on the baking sheet to cook for 20 minutes.
2. For dried figs: Cover them with boiling water to soften and drain.
3. Add all of the ingredients in a food processor and mix thoroughly.
4. The tapenade will keep in the fridge for about one week in an airtight container.

Sour Cream

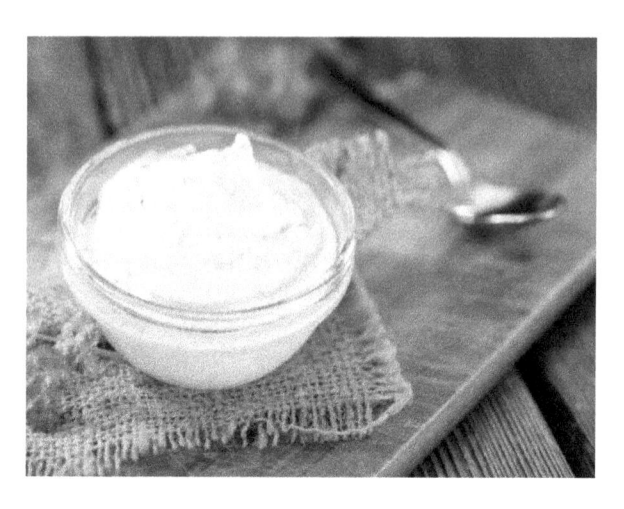

Makes: Little over 1 cup

Total preparation time: 5 min.

Ingredients:
- 1 c. of extra-firm silken or crumbled firm tofu
- 2-3 tbsp. of rice milk
- 2 tbsp. of lemon juice to taste
- ¼ t. of salt as desired

Directions:

1. Mix all of the ingredients in the blender or food processor. Purée until smooth.
2. Store in an airtight container.

Taco Seasoning

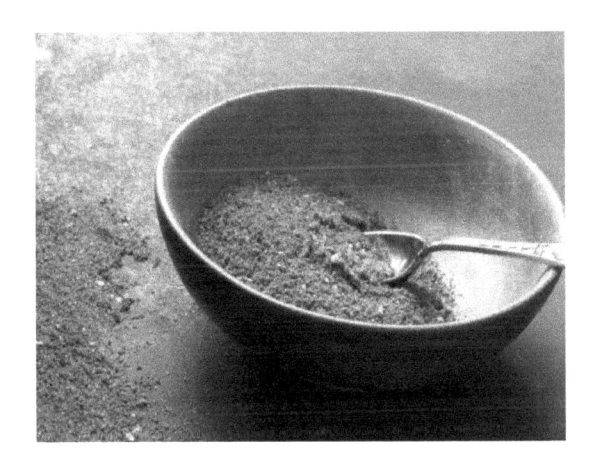

Makes: ¼ cup

Total preparation time: 5 min.
Ingredients:

- 2 t. of paprika
- ½ t. of garlic powder
- 3 t. of chili powder
- 1 t. of each:
- Ground coriander
- Dried oregano
- Ground cumin
- Black pepper
- Sea salt

Directions:

1. Simply whisk all of the ingredients of the seasoning together.
2. Cover and shake. If kept at room temperature, it will last for up to six months.
3. To change the flavor, add ½ tbsp. chipotle powder or an additional teaspoon of the garlic powder. It is all up to you!

White Bean Hummus

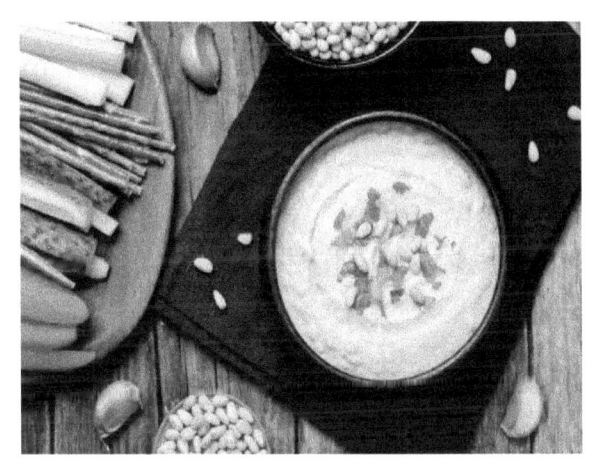

Makes: 6-8 servings

Total preparation time: 5 min.

Ingredients:
- 1 (15 oz.) can of cannellini beans
- 1-3 tbsp. of water
- 2 tbsp. of toasted sesame oil
- 1 t. of garlic powder
- ¼ t. of sea salt & ground black pepper
- ½ t. of ground cumin
- Olive oil to drizzle

Directions:
1. Rinse and drain the beans. Prepare with 1 tbsp. of water (to start), the sesame oil, salt, pepper, cumin, and garlic powder.
2. Mix until you reach the desired consistency, adding just a little water at a time.
3. Serve with a drizzle of oil.

Snacks

Banana Cookies

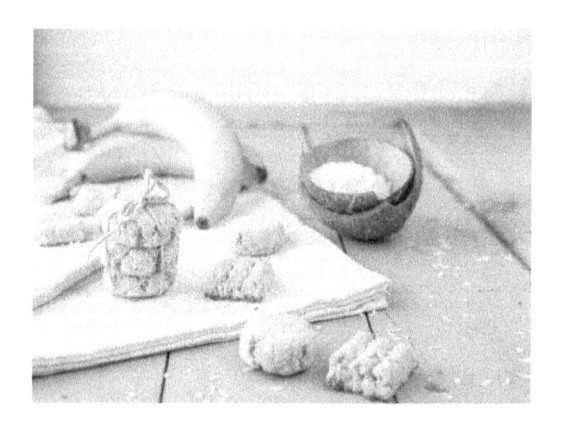

Makes: 36 servings
Total preparation time: 50 min.

Ingredients:
- 2 c. of rolled oats
- 3 ripened bananas
- 1/3 c. of vegetable oil
- 1 c. of dates
- 1 t. of vanilla extract

*Directions***:**
1. Pit and chop the dates. Set the oven's temperature to 350ºF.
2. Smash the bananas in a large bowl and add the rest of the ingredients.
3. Let the dough rest for 15 minutes. Scoop by teaspoon onto a cookie sheet.
4. Bake until browned, will take about 20 minutes.

Cashew & Dates Dessert

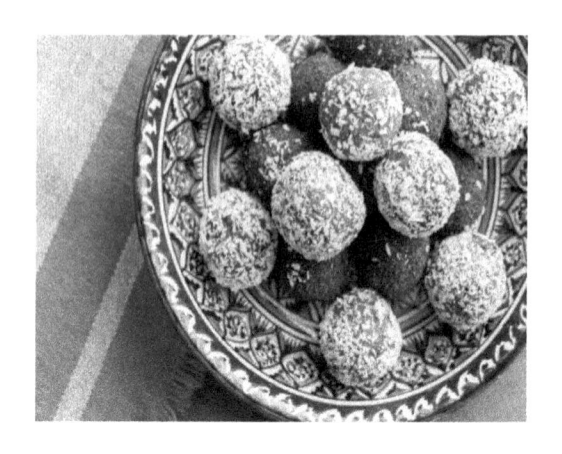

Makes: 20 servings

Total preparation time: 15 min.

Ingredients:
- 1 ¼ c. of raw cashews
- 1 c. of pitted dates
- Orange zest
- ½ c. of coconut flakes
- ¼ t. of cardamom

Directions:

1. Use a food processor to grind the dates, adding the cashews until finely ground. Whisk in the cardamom and zest.

2. Shape the dough into one-inch balls and sprinkle with some coconut flakes.

3. Serve and enjoy the yummy treats anytime.

Double-chocolate, Almond Chia Seed

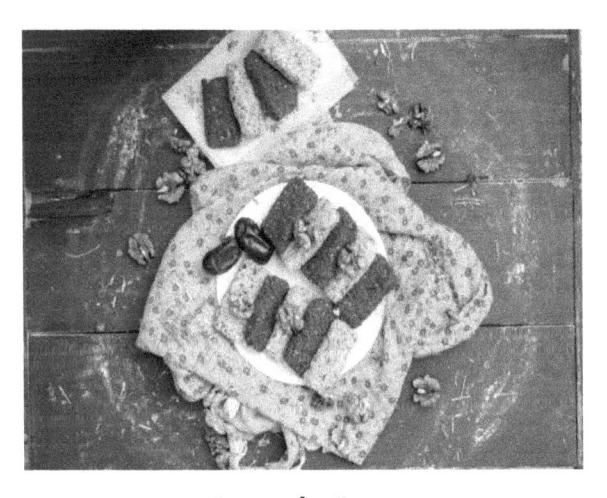

Granola Bars

Total preparation time: 28 min.

Makes: 8 servings

Ingredients:
- ½ c. of chocolate/vanilla protein powder
- 1 ¾ c. of old fashioned oats
- 1 t. of each:
- Cocoa powder
- Chia seeds
- ¼ c. of maple syrup
- 1 t. of cinnamon
- ½ c. of each:
- Natural peanut butter
- Unsweetened almond milk
- ¼ t. of salt
- 2 tbsp. of each:
- Mini chocolate chips
- Chopped almonds
- Sea salt for sprinkling

*Also needed***:** 9x9 baking pan

*Directions***:**

1. Set the oven to 350ºF. Lightly grease the baking pan.
2. Mix the protein powder, oats, cocoa powder, chia seeds, salt, and cinnamon.
3. In a smaller dish, microwave the maple and peanut butter for 30 seconds. Stir well and add to the oat mixture. Pour in the milk to form a soft dough.
4. Pour the dough into the pan and sprinkle the almonds, pressing them into the dough slightly. Bake until set for about 15-18 minutes.
5. Transfer to the counter, and sprinkle with the chocolate chips and salt.
6. Place them in the fridge until they're ready to eat.

Oatmeal Energy Bars

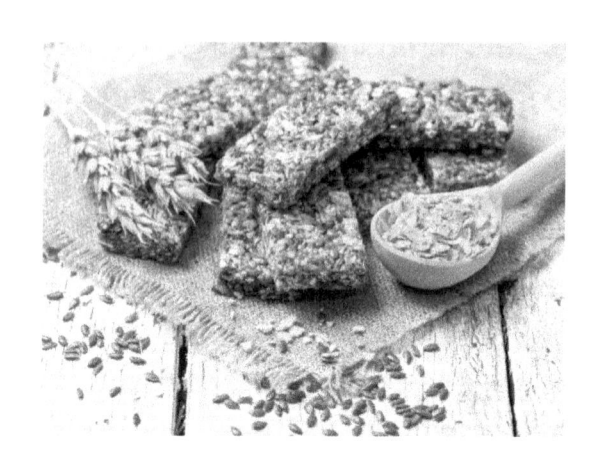

Makes: 24 servings

Total preparation time: 40 min.

Ingredients:
- ½ c. of each:
- All-purpose flour
- Unsalted Ground Cashews
- Vegan semi-sweet chocolate chips
- 1 1/3 c. of rolled oats
- 2 tbsp. of shelled and unsalted sunflower seeds
- 1 t. of each:

- Ground flax meal
- Wheat germ
- ¼ t. of sea salt
- ½ t. of each:
- Ground cinnamon
- Vanilla extract
- 1/3 c. of almond butter
- ½ c. of warmed maple syrup

Also needed: 9x11 baking dish

Directions:
1. Program the oven to 350ºF. Line the baking dish with foil.
2. Combine the sea salt, oats, chocolate chips, flour, cashews, sunflower seeds, wheat germ, and flax meal together in a shallow mixing dish. Blend in the vanilla, almond butter, and warmed syrup until well combined.
3. Empty the batter into the baking dish. Press firmly using a section of the wax paper to flatten the mixture.

4. Bake for ten minutes, cover with foil and cool in the foil for ten minutes. Cut into bars.

Appetizers

Mushroom Bruschetta Crostini

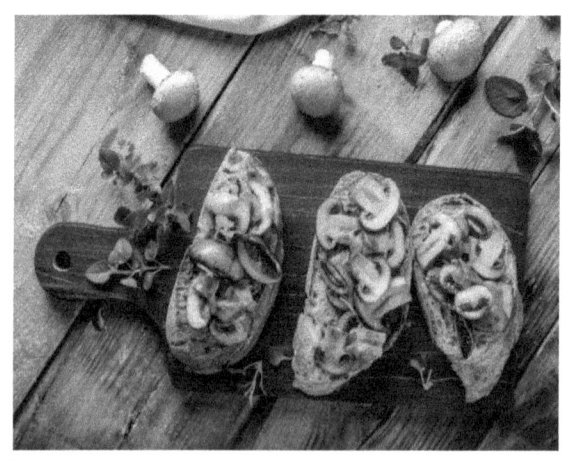

Makes: 36 crostini

Total preparation time: 30 minutes

Ingredients:
- ½ c. of diced onion

- 2 tbsp. of extra-virgin olive oil or coconut oil
- 1 diced red bell pepper
- 8 oz. of *cremini* mushrooms
- ¼ t. of black pepper
- ½ t. of sea salt
- 1 long loaf of Italian bread

Directions:

1. Warm up the oil in a skillet. Sauté the peppers and onions for ten minutes. Blend in the mushrooms and sauté for another 10-15 minutes.
2. Flavor with a shake of pepper and salt.
3. Make the crostini by slicing the baguette. Brush each of the slices with oil. Place them on the cookie sheet. Broil them for several minutes.
4. Remove when golden and spoon on the bruschetta.
5. Garnish as you choose.

White Bean Bruschetta

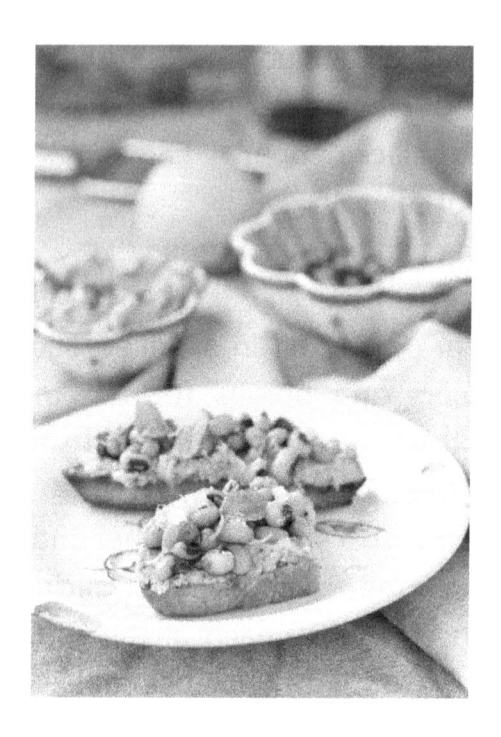

Makes: 4-6 servings

Total preparation time: 10 min.

Ingredients:
- 3 plum tomatoes
- 1 can (15 oz.) of cannellini beans
- 1 garlic clove

- 2 tbsp. of olive oil
- ¼ c. of Kalamata olives
- ¼ c. of chopped fresh basil
- ¼ t. each of salt and pepper
- 1 baguette, sliced into ½-inch thickness

Directions:
1. Remove the seeds and chop the tomatoes. Rinse and drain the beans. Also, chop the olives and garlic to bits.
2. Combine all of the ingredients until well incorporated.
3. Add a spoonful to a toasted baguette, slice, and enjoy!

Chapter 6: Desserts

Pumpkin & Apple Dessert

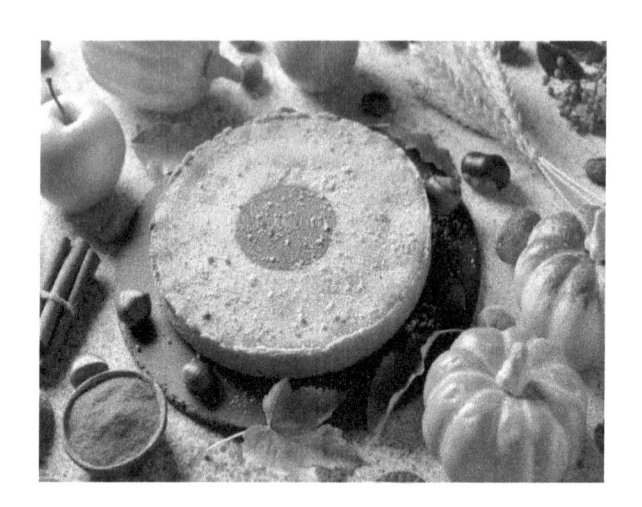

Makes: 1 serving

Total preparation time: 9 min.

Ingredients:
- 2 packs or 1 g. of sugar substitute
- 1 Granny Smith apple
- 1 t. of pumpkin pie spice
- 2 tbsp. of water

- ¼ c. of canned pumpkin

Also needed: Microwavable dish

Directions:
1. Empty 1/3 teaspoon pumpkin spice and 1/3 package of the sugar substitute into the bottom of a mixing container. Layer ¼ of the apples in the bowl, adding the pumpkin over the apples. Add the rest of the sugar substitute and spice to the mix.
2. Toss in the rest of the apples and empty the water over the contents.
3. Cook in the microwave for 3 ½ minutes, stirring at one-minute intervals.
4. Serve when ready.

Pumpkin Bread

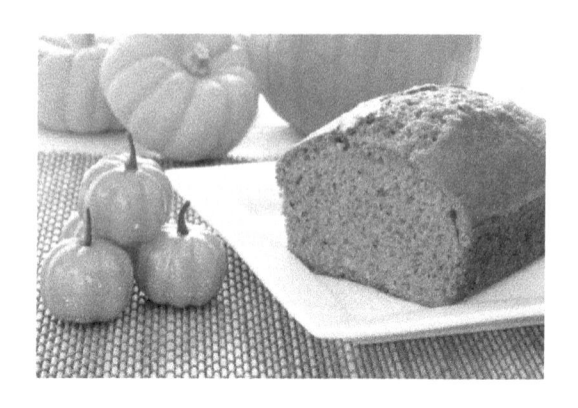

Makes: 3 loaves

Total preparation time: 1 hr. and 5 min.

Ingredients:
- 2/3 c. of water
- 4 eggs
- 1 can (15 oz.) of pumpkin purée
- 1 ½ c. of molasses, equal to 3 c. of white sugar
- 1 tbsp. of each:
- Cinnamon
- Nutmeg
- 3 ½ c. of all-purpose flour

- 1 ½ tbsp. of salt
- ½ tbsp. of ground cloves
- ¼ tbsp. of ground ginger
- 2 of tbsp. of baking soda
- 1 c. of canola oil

*Also need*ed: 3 (7x3-inch) loaf pans

Directions:
1. Heat the oven to 350ºF.
2. Lightly grease and add flour to the loaf pans. Shake out the excess flour and make sure you covered the entire pan with the oil.
3. Use a large mixing container to mix the sugar, water, oil, puree, and eggs until blended well.
4. In another container, mix the ginger, cloves, cinnamon, flour, nutmeg, baking soda, and salt.
5. Mix all of the ingredients until well-blended and add to the loaf pans.
6. Bake for 50 minutes.

Raw Strawberry Pie

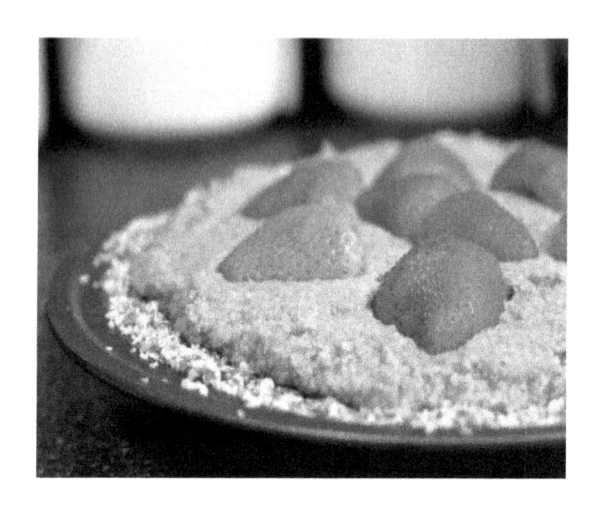

Makes: 10 servings

Total preparation time: 2 hrs. 20 min.

Ingredients (Step 1):
- 1 pinch of salt
- 2 t. of coconut oil
- 1 c. of each:
- Pitted dates
- Shredded coconut
- Almonds

Ingredients (Step 3):
- 2 c. of each:
- Shredded coconut
- Strawberries
- 2 t. of coconut oil
- 1 pinch of salt
- 3 sliced strawberries

Directions:
1. Add all of the ingredients in this step, from the salt to the almonds.
2. Arrange the dough into the pan and form the crust.
3. Add the rest of the ingredients listed for this step in a blender. Purée until it's creamy.
4. Pour the cream over the crust, followed by the berries. Place in the fridge for about two hours until the pie thickens.

Smoothies

Banana Pineapple & Nutty Smoothie

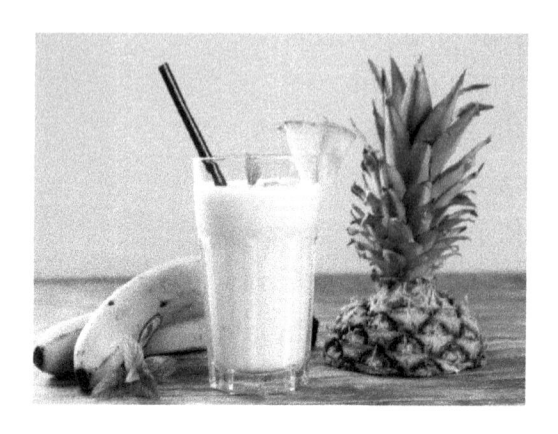

Makes: 2 servings

Total preparation time: 10 minutes

Ingredients:
- 1 c. pineapple chunks
- 2 bananas
- 2 tbsp. of each:
- Chopped walnuts
- Cashew butter
- 2 c. water

Directions:
1. Combine the walnuts, butter, pineapple, and bananas in a blender.
2. Pour in some water until the mixture becomes smooth.

Blueberry & Lemonade Smoothie

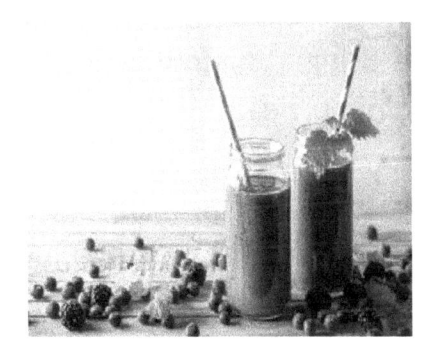

Makes: 1 serving

Total preparation time: 5 min.

Ingredients:
- ¾ c. of frozen blueberries
- 1 c. each of:
- Roughly chopped kale

- Unsweetened soy/almond milk
- 1 tbsp. of maple syrup
- Juice of 1 lemon

Variations:
- **Tropical smoothie**

  Use ½ cup (each) of mango chunks and pineapple chunks.

- **Lemonade strawberry smoothie**

  Prepare using 1 c. strawberries instead of the blueberries.

Directions:
1. Combine all of the ingredients in a blender. Mix until smooth and creamy.
2. Serve in a chilled glass and relax!

Cherry Smoothie

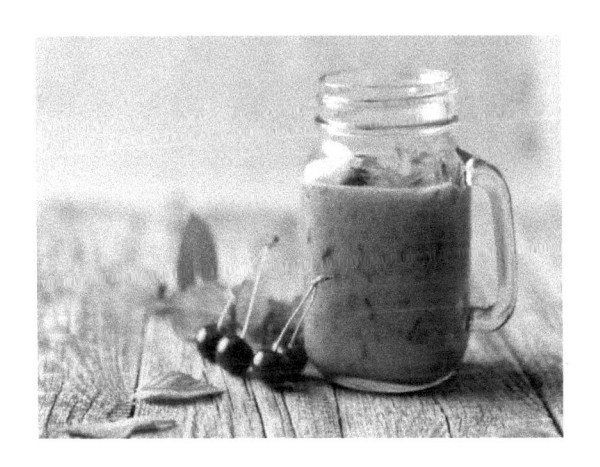

Makes: 2 servings

Total preparation time: 7 min.

Ingredients:
- 2 med-large ripened bananas, this is better frozen
- 2 c. of frozen tart cherries
- 1 c. of coconut water or plain water
- 1 t. of almond or vanilla extract
- Stevia or agave to taste

Directions:
1. Mix everything in a blender until it becomes creamy.
2. Serve right away and enjoy!

Chia Banana & Green Tea Smoothie

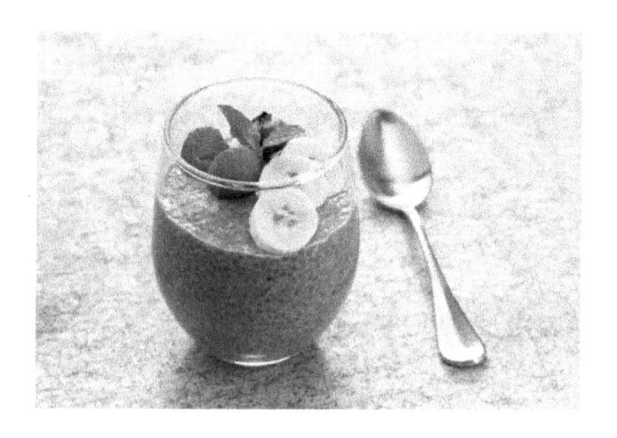

Makes: 1 serving

Total preparation time: 6 min.

Ingredients:
- 1 med. banana, frozen or not
- ½ tbsp. of *matcha* green tea powder

- 1 ½ t. of almond milk
- 1 tbsp. of chia seeds
- 1 scoop of stevia powder extract or a pkg. of Swerve

Directions:
1. Add all of the ingredients and pulse until creamy.
2. You can add ice cubes if the bananas are not frozen.
3. Let it sit for one minute for the chia to thicken.

Matcha Coconut Smoothie

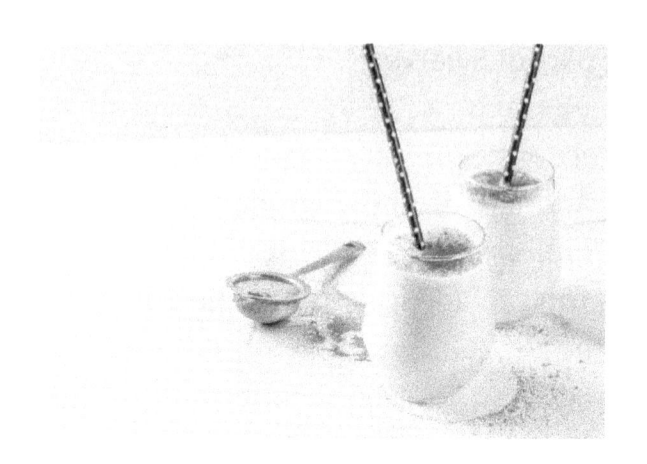

Makes: 1 serving

Total preparation time: 10 min.

Ingredients:
- 1 c. of frozen mango chunks
- 1 banana
- 2 kale leaves
- 3 tbsp. of drained white beans
- ½ t. of *matcha* green tea powder

- 2 tbsp. of unsweetened, shredded coconut
- 1 c. of water

Directions:
1. Tear the kale into several pieces and add the remainder of the ingredients.
2. Blend until the mixture becomes creamy smooth.

Orange Juice Goji Berries Smoothie

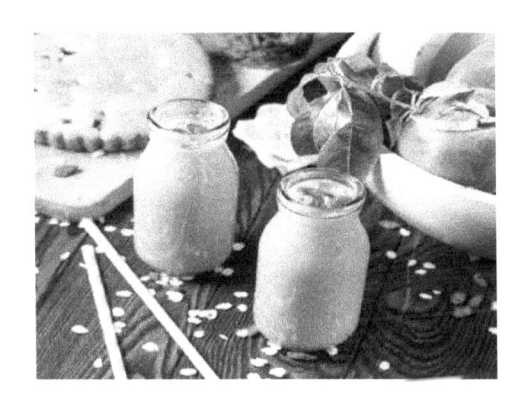

Makes: 1 serving

Total preparation time: 5 min.

Ingredients:
- 2 slices of fresh ginger
- 1 tbsp. of goji berries
- 1 c. of freshly squeezed orange juice

Directions:
1. Blend the ginger, berries, and juice in a blender until it's puréed.
2. Pour and enjoy.

Conclusion

Thanks for reading your entire copy of the *book*. Let's hope it was informative and that it provided you with all of the tools you need to achieve your goals whatever they may be.

The next step is to prepare a list of guidelines using your favorite recipes. Surely, you must have found at least four or five you want to try right away.

About the Author

Kenny Brown is author of several cookbooks on vegan diet. He has written research papers on the topic and currently lives in California.